D1136764

LIBRARY

Reproductive Technology

Other titles in the series:

Information Technology and Cyberspace: Extra-connected Living
by David Pullinger

Forthcoming titles include:

Punishment
by Christopher Jones

Human Genetics
by Robert Song

Euthanasia
by Nigel Biggar

Reproductive Technology

Towards a Theology of
Procreative Stewardship

BRENT WATERS

DARTON·LONGMAN + TODD

First published in 2001 by
Darton, Longman and Todd Ltd
1 Spencer Court
140–142 Wandsworth High Street
London SW18 4JJ

ISBN 0-232-52360-6

A catalogue record for this book is available from the British Library.

Designed by Sandie Boccacci
Phototypeset in 10/13 $^1/_4$pt Palatino by Intype London Ltd
Printed and bound in Great Britain by
The Cromwell Press, Trowbridge, Wiltshire

Contents

vi   Contents

Acknowledgements

SIGNIFICANT PORTIONS of this book are adapted from my D.Phil. thesis at the University of Oxford. I am indebted to my supervisor, Oliver O'Donovan, for his wise and patient guidance. In addition, I would like to thank the Committee of Vice-Chancellors and Principals of the Universities of the United Kingdom (CVCP) for granting me an Overseas Research Student Award while studying at Oxford. I also want to express my gratitude to my editor at Darton, Longman and Todd, Katie Worrall, not only for envisioning this project but also for keeping me focused and on schedule. Finally, the love and support of my wife, Diana, and daughter, Erin, have once again provided a great source of strength and inspiration.

Introduction

TO AN UNPRECEDENTED EXTENT, we may now control or intervene in the human reproductive process. A variety of techniques assist conception or fertilisation. A pregnant woman can carry a fetus with whom she shares no genetic connection. Fetuses are monitored for a wide range of illnesses and disabilities. Embryos may be tested for a growing number of debilitating conditions. Reproductive technology has become very much a part of contemporary life.

These technological developments, however, are accompanied by some troubling moral questions: does a person have a right to reproduce? Does an embryo or fetus have a right to life? Is marriage, or other committed relationships, weakened by the use of donated gametes or embryos? Is a parent–child relationship primarily a biological or social bond? Are children affected adversely by multiple or unknown parentage? Do parents have a right to prevent the birth of ill or disabled offspring? Or more broadly: does the advent of reproductive technology transgress lines of natural and moral limits that we cross at our peril? Or to the contrary: is our growing ability to control our propagation unleashing a creative potential to construct a more humane world?

Given these types of questions, it is not surprising that theologians have produced a voluminous literature on reproductive technology. These assessments range from a virtual repudiation of any artificial intervention to nearly carte blanche endorsement, while most positions lie somewhere in between. What is rarely given much explicit attention, however, is how the theological convictions of these writers inform their disparate moral assessments.

The purpose of this book is to portray how Christian

theological convictions may be used in constructing moral arguments on a number of selected issues. The intent is not to defend the Christian position on each of these issues, but rather to depict how certain theological convictions shape an author's moral argument. Moreover, the primary objective is not to persuade readers that the positions presented here are necessarily the best ones, but to invite them to engage in their own theologically informed process of moral deliberation on questions raised by reproductive technology.

Yet it should not be assumed that this book is a dispassionate exercise. I believe the positions I argue for are true, but defending their veracity is a secondary, rather than primary, goal. This approach is adopted to counter two prevailing trends. On the one hand, a particular position is argued by ignoring or dismissing alternative stances, while on the other hand, various positions are summarised but the reader is given no indication which option the author prefers. The former approach fails to indicate where a particular position fits within a range of options, while the latter fails to suggest how or why some positions may be judged to be better than others. In emphasising how certain theological convictions shape a pattern of moral deliberation, I hope to demonstrate where the positions I favour fit within a range of attitudes, and why or on what basis I contend they are preferable to their alternatives.

To initiate this approach, the first chapter provides an overview of various reproductive technologies, as well as a critical summary of the dominant moral framework in which they are assessed. It argues that as humans exert greater control over the reproductive process, a sense of mystery is being displaced by one of mastery. This shift is seen in what is described as the 'medicalisation' of procreation. The deployment of various techniques is creating an expanding range of reproductive options. A once presumed continuity between procreation and child-rearing is carved into a series of discrete tasks involving conception, gestation, birth and 'parenting'.

This fragmentation of procreation and child-rearing reflects moral presuppositions that are characterised as 'procreative

liberty'. The central tenet is that since each person has a fundamental interest in either avoiding or pursuing reproduction,
then every person also has a right to use those techniques which
best assist them in pursuing their reproductive interests. A
medicalised pursuit of procreation helps individuals achieve
their reproductive goals. Thus few restrictions should be placed
on reproductive technologies, because they enlarge the scope
of one's personal freedom.

The principal complaint against this moral framework is its
excessive individualism. In fixating on the reproductive
interests and rights of individuals, a larger network of biological
and social relationships impinging upon the moral ordering of
procreation and child-rearing are virtually ignored. Consequently, procreative liberty fails to address a number of
significant moral considerations. Given these limitations, an
alternative moral framework is needed.

Chapter 2 provides a theological foundation for this alternative framework by examining four themes.

1. Life is a gift and loan from God, and humans, in particular,
    are creatures bearing God's image and likeness. Since
    humans belong to God, they should not treat themselves
    or others as possessions or property.
2. A dualistic understanding of persons, as often presumed
    by advocates of procreative liberty, is incompatible with
    our status as God's creatures. Humans are not creatures
    composed of a body *and* a soul. Rather, God has created us
    as embodied souls and ensouled bodies. Moreover, our
    life as persons unfolds within and through covenants com-
    prising both biological and social bonds.
3. Marriage provides a normative foundation for a familial
    covenant of mutual love and fidelity that is oriented toward
    the procreation and rearing of children. Within this
    covenant, children do not belong to their parents but to
    God who entrusts them to the care of parents. As a cov-
    enant, however, the family requires a moral ordering of its
    biological and social bonds, especially in respect to

procreation and child-rearing. In short, parenthood cannot be reduced to either biology or a social construct.

4. The moral ordering of procreation and child-rearing requires a stewardship of the familial covenant. Thus reproductive technologies may be assessed by whether they tend to enable or disable the stewardship of this covenant. The principal consideration in making this judgement is whether or not a particular application of a reproductive technology tends to honour or violate the standards of life as gift and loan, of embodied personhood, and of the integrity of familial relationships.

The following chapters refine this theological framework by exploring the issues of childlessness and parenthood, preventing and assisting reproduction, and quality control and experimentation. Chapter 3 examines the reasons why people may want to have children. The chapter begins with an overview of biblical and historical sources. Whereas the Old Testament tends to portray offspring as a blessing and childlessness as a curse, the New Testament relativises the significance of procreation, parenthood and lineage. Subsequent developments in Christian thinking are also examined. Against this biblical and historical background, a number of contemporary positions on the extent to which the parent–child relationship is defined by a biological bond are summarised. These positions range from an absolute necessity for this bond to its total irrelevance.

In placing my argument within this range, I contend that although a biological bond is a significant element in a normative understanding of parenthood, it is not the overriding factor. Rather, the most pressing consideration is entrusting children to the care of parents. Children and parents are bound together in a covenant of mutual belonging, love and fidelity. Although this covenant often includes a biological bond between parent and child, it does not preclude a calling to the parental vocation through such non-procreative means as adoption or foster care. This position, however, leaves an important question unresolved: may reproductive technologies be employed to assist persons in fulfilling their calling to the parental vocation?

In addressing this question, the next chapter examines to what extent humans may intervene in natural processes to assist or prevent procreation. The context for this investigation is the recent debate on contraception and collaborative reproduction involving artificial insemination, donated gametes, *in vitro* fertilisation, and surrogacy. Once again representative positions are summarised, ranging from a complete prohibition of any artificial intervention to libertarian views permitting virtually any intervention.

Given the scope of these options, I argue that our status as embodied creatures offers a normative pattern for how pro-creation should be pursued, but is not the sole criterion. The covenantal considerations of mutual belonging, love and fidelity must also be taken into account. Thus I contend that contraception, artificial insemination and *in vitro* fertilisation (not employing donated gametes) do not sufficiently distort the embodied or covenantal qualities of procreation to proscribe their use. Once again, however, this position does not resolve a significant issue: if it is permissible to assist natural repro-ductive processes, may techniques be employed to control the qualitative outcomes of procreation?

The final chapter explores the extent to which reproductive technologies may be employed to prevent the birth of a child with a severely deleterious disease or disability. Although it is understandable that parents want to have healthy offspring, does this desire justify destroying embryos or fetuses when such 'quality-control' techniques as fetal monitoring, embryo testing and selective implantation are deployed? In addition, may experiments be conducted on embryos to further scientific knowledge? As in the previous two chapters, representative positions are summarised, ranging from prohibiting all quality-control techniques and experimentation to few, if any, restrictions.

In placing my position within this range I concede that a routine employment of quality-control techniques would jeopardise the unconditional character of the familial covenant. Parental affection might be withheld until a fetus or embryo 'passes' certain tests. Parental care, however, includes a responsibility to promote the health of offspring that may be expressed at the antenatal level. Within carefully proscribed diagnostic parameters such a technique as testing and selectively implanting embryos is permissible if the intent is to prevent the birth of a child with a severely deleterious disease or disability. In addition, I contend that research may be conducted on affected embryos if the purpose is to develop therapies for treating the deleterious condition that a technique is employed to prevent.

As the discussions of these issues will demonstrate, reproductive technology lends itself to examining how theological convictions inform moral deliberation. Our growing ability to assert greater control over how life is transmitted from one generation to the next touches on many of the core beliefs of Christian faith. In light of our growing capability to manipulate the earliest stages of human life, what does it mean to be creatures created in the image and likeness of God? What is required of us as creatures bearing this image? Do these new technologies help or hinder us in exercising our stewardship of the gift and loan of life entrusted to us by God?

Even if most of us are never affected directly by a particular reproductive technology, their presence nonetheless alters our lives. The advent of reproductive technology has changed, and will continue to change, how we perceive procreation and how it should be pursued. As Marilyn Strathern has written: 'These technologies can be considered as instruments of change themselves, indeed as already having caused change in the way people think about the reproductive process.'[1]

If we are starting to think differently about procreation, about what it means to be a child or a parent, then it is incumbent upon us to be careful about how this thinking shapes, for good or ill, our moral discernment. This is the point where theology plays a central role, for it provides the base and pattern of our discernment. It is not so much the case that our ethics force us to change our beliefs, but rather that faith is the content of our ethics. The purpose of moral deliberation is, after all, to make us wise rather than clever. We may very well formulate clever policies governing the uses of reproductive technology without ever broaching the question of whether these uses are good or wise. A process of moral deliberation alone cannot make this determination. Rather, it is the truth and strength of the convictions that moral arguments seek to clarify and expound that make us wise rather than clever.

This does not suggest that new scientific and technological developments should not inspire fresh theological accounts of Christian faith. Christian theology does not presume to know everything about the faith it seeks to understand, nor everything about the created order in which it seeks understanding. Rather, theology helps us discern puzzling reflections in a mirror; we see but only in part.[2] As Christians we should not be too hasty either to condemn or to commend reproductive technology. We must first turn to our faith to gain some clarity of conviction on what confronts us, and how we should respond to this power over the beginning of human lives that is now at our disposal.

chapter one

Reproductive Options

This chapter provides an overview of various reproductive technologies, as well as a critical summary of the dominant moral framework in which they are assessed. The first section describes currently available techniques, and is followed by an examination of the medicalisation of procreation. The concluding sections assess the adequacy of the dominant moral framework that is portrayed as 'procreative liberty', with its heavy emphasis upon the interests and rights of autonomous persons.

THE BIRTH OF THE WORLD'S first 'test-tube baby' in 1978 may be used to mark the beginning of a new era of reproductive technology. Louise Brown was the first baby to be born using *in vitro* fertilisation. Although techniques assisting reproduction pre-date this event, never before had a child been born who was conceived outside of a woman's womb. This unprecedented achievement has spurred a series of rapid developments in reproductive technology, forming in its wake a widening range of moral concerns. This chapter examines how these developments are altering our perception of procreation, as well as the dominant framework in which the ethical issues accompanying them are perceived and assessed.

From procreative mystery to reproductive management

The Psalmist extols God:

> For it was you who formed my inward parts;
>   you knit me together in my mother's womb.
> I praise you, for I am fearfully and wonderfully made.
>   Wonderful are your works;
>   that I know very well.
> My frame was not hidden from you,
>   when I was being made in secret,
>   intricately woven in the depths of the earth.[1]

These words capture the mystery that has enveloped procreation throughout much of human history. Transmitting life from one generation to the next involved powerful forces beyond the understanding of humans and, much more, beyond their control and manipulation. Through the secret workings of the body, it was God who formed and brought into being a new child, God alone who chose to open or close a woman's womb.

In the face of such power it is not surprising that the Psalmist responded with a sense of awe, wonder and fear. There was little humans could do, for instance, to overcome infertility or control the characteristics of offspring. Although unreliable techniques have been employed in the past, they were largely ineffective in asserting greater control over this mysterious power. It was only after, rather than before, birth that parents could play a more active role.

Unlike the Psalmist we no longer believe that God's weaving-in-the-womb, so to speak, is hidden from our view. We know much more about human biology in general and reproduction in particular. This knowledge may be applied in asserting greater control over what was once believed to be a mysterious power beyond our comprehension. In short, a sense of procreative mystery is giving way to one of reproductive management. Moreover, the range of reproductive technologies at our disposal enables us to assert this managerial control more expansively and efficiently.

Various techniques have been developed to overcome physiological factors preventing conception or fertilisation. These technologies are often referred to collectively as *assisted reproductive technologies* or ART. The most prevalent causes of infertility include tubal factors, endometriosis, ovulatory dysfunction, and male sterility or low sperm count. The oldest technique is *artificial insemination* (AI) in which semen is injected into a woman's vagina or uterus, with sperm provided by the husband (AIH) or a donor (AID).

In vitro fertilisation (IVF) involves fertilising an egg in a laboratory and transferring the embryo into a woman's uterus through the cervix. Normally two or three embryos are transferred with the hope that at least one will implant resulting in a pregnancy and live birth.

Two techniques employed less frequently are *gamete intrafallopian transfer* (GIFT) and *zygote intrafallopian transfer* (ZIFT). In the former technique, a laparoscope (a small optical instrument that is inserted into the pelvic cavity) is used to place eggs and sperm in the fallopian tubes through tiny incisions in the abdomen. In the latter instance, a laparoscope is used to place fertilised eggs or zygotes in the fallopian tubes.

In each instance, spouses or donors may provide the gametes. In addition, excess gametes and embryos may be frozen and used in subsequent cycles if the first attempt fails or if additional children are wanted at a later date. The success rate (number of live births per 100 cycles) ranges from 9.6 per cent to 21.8 per cent depending on such factors as the technique employed, whether fresh or frozen gametes or embryos are used, and the age of the woman. In comparison with natural reproduction it is estimated that somewhere between 30 per cent and 70 per cent of zygotes either fail to implant, or a pregnancy ends in a spontaneous abortion, miscarriage or stillbirth.[2]

Although *surrogacy* is being used increasingly, it is not a new technique. In the Old Testament, for instance, a younger brother could have sexual intercourse with his older brother's childless widow to perpetuate the older brother's lineage.[3] ART, however, makes a variety of surrogacy arrangements possible. A surrogate may be artificially inseminated, and following birth the man providing the sperm and his infertile wife or partner adopt the child. In this case the child is genetically related to her father and surrogate mother, but not to her social mother. Or a couple may not be infertile but the woman is unable to maintain a pregnancy. Using IVF, embryos are placed in a surrogate. In this instance the child is genetically related to both of her social parents but not to the woman who bore her. Or a couple may use donated gametes (usually eggs) for the IVF cycle and place the zygotes in a surrogate. In this case the child is not genetically related to one (and possibly none) of her social parents, or to the surrogate mother.

ART may also be employed to 'treat' conditions or circumstances other than infertility. These techniques may assist single persons or individuals without appropriate partners to become parents. A single man, for example, may employ AI or IVF and a surrogate, or a lesbian couple could use donated sperm and IVF to implant the fertilised eggs or zygotes of one partner in the other. *Posthumous reproduction* is now possible. A widow, for instance, may be impregnated with the frozen sperm of her dead husband, or a widower could have the frozen embryos he and his wife had produced earlier implanted in a surrogate. Post-menopausal women have been assisted in becoming pregnant, and young women may freeze their eggs to use at a later date, lowering the risk of chromosomal abnormalities. If reproductive *cloning* becomes feasible in the future then the genome of a living or dead person may be replicated. An infertile man with the aid of donated eggs and a surrogate could clone himself to have a son to whom he is genetically related, or grieving parents could clone their dead or dying child.

In addition to assisting reproduction we may now assert greater *quality control* over reproductive outcomes. All too often the natural reproductive process goes awry, resulting in severely debilitating illnesses and disabilities. In order to

produce healthier offspring, as well as spare parents the heart-
ache and burden of caring for severely ill or disabled children,
we may either *prevent* a range of undesirable traits, or *select*
desirable ones. Although such unreliable quality-control techniques as mate selection, sterilisation and infanticide have been
used in the past, we now have at our disposal more reliable,
as well as presumably more humane, methods for ensuring or
maximising the health of children.

A number of techniques, known collectively as *prenatal diagnosis* (PND), may be employed to monitor or test fetal
development. *Ultrasound imaging* passes sound waves through a
pregnant woman's body. The resulting 'sonogram' can disclose
obvious physical features or abnormalities of a fetus, as well
as other potential problems associated with pregnancy. More
sophisticated techniques include *amniocentesis* and *chorionic
villus sampling* (CVS). The former technique involves inserting
a needle into the uterus to withdraw amniotic fluid,[4] while the
latter involves inserting a needle into the abdomen to remove
chorionic villi (hair-like material) from the placenta.[5] In both
instances fetal cells are tested for chromosomal or genetic
abnormalities.

Although these techniques can be employed to identify an
expanding range of deleterious traits, they incorporate several
liabilities. Ultrasound imaging can only disclose a limited range
of physical features, while amniocentesis and CVS subject both
mother and fetus to relatively small degrees of risk. Furthermore, although the accuracy of these tests is improving, their
reliability is limited, nor can the severity of a deleterious trait
be predicted in many instances. Since most of the conditions
diagnosed cannot be treated *in utero*, the only options parents
have are to prepare themselves to care for an ill or disabled
child, or terminate the pregnancy.

A method for avoiding this dilemma, especially for individuals with a high risk of passing on deleterious traits to
offspring, is to employ *pre-implantation genetic diagnosis* (PGD).
One or two cells are removed from an embryo (created through
IVF), and a biopsy is performed to determine if the embryo is

affected by or carries certain deleterious genetic traits. Following these tests unaffected embryos are implanted in the uterus. Again, these tests are highly accurate but not foolproof, nor can severity be predicted in many cases. In addition, unaffected embryos are sometimes damaged during testing, or an inadequate number of unaffected embryos are created, resulting a lower live birth rate when IVF is used in conjunction with PGD. Nonetheless, PGD gives parents greater certitude that their offspring will be spared a debilitating illness or disability.

As this brief overview demonstrates, humans may now exert unprecedented control over their reproduction. We have at our disposal a growing assortment of reproductive options. We may choose different methods of conception or fertilisation, and we may select the eggs, sperm or embryos that provide the best prospect for healthy offspring. Infertility is no longer a barrier preventing procreation, and the parental fear of giving birth to a severely ill or disabled child is being reduced. Although admittedly our control over the reproductive process and its outcomes remains limited, it is likely that future technological developments will push these limits back even further. We are no longer hapless observers of a procreative mystery but are becoming reproductive managers.

Asserting such managerial control, however, requires that parents not be left to their own devices. They must turn increasingly to medicine to exercise their reproductive options, for deploying the suitable technologies requires a requisite skill and expertise. There are no 'over-the-counter' products for performing IVF or PGD at home. Yet is this growing role of medicine altering our perception of how procreation should be pursued and what parenthood is coming to mean?

The medicalisation of procreation

According to Michael Burgess, *medicalisation* denotes a changing perception of a situation or set of circumstances from 'individual misfortune or a community nuisance' to that of a

'diagnosed condition'. Thus medicalisation 'confers legiti-
mation of the problem, social resources for research into causes
and treatment, and often a different configuration of responsibility'.[6] As reproductive technology is more widely deployed,
procreation in turn becomes medicalised.

Specifically, the misfortune of *childlessness* is transformed into
the problem of *infertility*. Infertility, unlike childlessness, is a
medical condition that can be 'treated'. Likewise, the misfortune
and nuisance of caring for severely ill or disabled children
is transformed into the problem of preventing unnecessary
illness and suffering. Treating infertility and preventing illness
justifies large investments in developing and delivering
more effective technologies, enabling individuals to assume
greater responsibility for pursuing their reproductive interests
and ensuring the health of offspring. We are no longer passive
'victims' of infertility or reproductive processes gone awry,
but may take action to correct or prevent these undesirable
circumstances.

Reproductive technology has undoubtedly helped many
infertile people become parents, and prevented the birth of a
number of children who would otherwise endure debilitating
pain and suffering. This same technology, however, promotes
and reinforces a changing perception that may be described as
an *emerging pattern of procreation and child-rearing*. There is a
widening spectrum of options for how offspring may be
brought into being, ranging from sexual intercourse to complex
collaborative arrangements involving IVF, donated gametes,
surrogacy and embryo screening. This emerging pattern displaces continuity through marriage, procreation and
parenthood by dividing conception, gestation and child-rearing
into a series of discrete tasks.

Sexual intercourse is increasingly separated from marriage. This
division obviously pre-dates the advent of reproductive technology as perennial prohibitions against fornication, adultery
and incest attest. Recent cultural changes and technological
developments, however, are altering prevalent mores concerning sexual conduct. Easy access to contraception and

abortion has lessened the prospect of unwanted children, and it is often presumed that sexual experimentation plays a crucial role in forming a person's identity. Repressing a person's sexual expression by requiring continent singleness, or restricting it to monogamous marriage, may retard or harm an individual's development. Consequently, separating sexual intercourse from procreation expedites personal well-being, requiring the construction of a more relevant sexual ethic.[7]

Procreation is increasingly separated from sexual intercourse. This is due not only to contraception, but also to the fact that coitus is now one reproductive option among many. AI and IVF, for example, may be employed not only by infertile couples, but also by individuals for whom sexual intercourse is an undesirable or unavailable option. As indicated earlier, a lesbian or gay couple, a widow possessing the frozen sperm of her dead husband, or an individual without a willing partner may use various reproductive options.

Parenthood is increasingly separated from procreation. Gamete donation and surrogacy are forcing reassessments of what parenthood signifies, requiring such qualifying prefixes as 'biological', 'carrying' or 'social' to designate a person's role in conception, gestation, birth and child-rearing. There are no objective standards defining parenthood. Although kinship is admittedly a social construct, traditional moral and legal codes attempted to delineate responsibilities incumbent upon relationships associated with a common bloodline. Natural parents may at times be unable or unwilling to perform their duties but they are nonetheless acknowledged, unlike anonymous gamete donors, as progenitors of a new life. As parenthood is carved into a series of discrete tasks, procreation is changed from an unfolding familial relationship into various reproductive tasks. Consequently, explicating the legal status and moral duties of parents requires a fundamental appraisal of the extent to which biology or biography defines what parenthood now means. Marilyn Strathern has stated the dilemma well:

The more we give legal certainty to social parenthood, the more we cut from under our feet assumptions about the intrinsic relationships themselves. The more facilitation is given to the biological reproduction of human persons, the harder it is to think of a domain of natural facts independent of social intervention.[8]

Child-rearing is increasingly separated from parenthood. This separation involves more than the perplexing challenge of defining parenthood when techniques such as gamete donation and surrogacy are employed. Rather, it reflects the ability to manipulate the reproductive process in line with parental goals regarding the kind of children that are wanted. As mentioned above, procreation no longer implies a biological process in which parents, up to the point of birth, play a relatively passive role. They may now intervene at various stages in obtaining a desirable, or avoiding an undesirable, outcome. A couple carrying a deleterious genetic trait, for example, may employ donated gametes, embryo screening and selective implantation, or fetal monitoring and abortion to prevent their offspring from being affected. In short, quality-control techniques give pregnancy and parenthood a provisional character.[9]

Two observations may be made regarding this emerging pattern. First, there is no normative structure ordering how procreation and child-rearing should be pursued. Rather, obtaining a child is a project in which such concerns as conception and gestation are intermediate and instrumental objectives. The ordering of procreation and child-rearing consists of matching ends and means, for no parental continuity, extending from conception through pregnancy, birth and child-rearing, is assumed. If a couple, for instance, want a child and encounter obstacles in achieving this goal, they face a series of choices: what method of conception should be employed? Whose gametes should be used or avoided? Whose body should provide gestation and give birth? To what extent should embryos be screened and fetuses monitored? Given the absence of an objective normative framework, there are no common standards for making these decisions. The suitability of each intermediate objective is determined by the overriding goal of obtaining a child, and reproductive technology is a means of pursuing one's desires.

Second, this emerging pattern presupposes a medicalised pursuit of procreation in which biological constraints and social roles are rendered largely irrelevant. Dividing procreation into a series of discrete tasks enables medicine to deploy reproductive technologies maximising a person's managerial control in achieving a desired goal or outcome. Moreover, a medicalised approach ignores or undercuts the familial roles and relationships traditionally associated with procreation and child-rearing, because a 'parent' is not necessarily a participant in each intermediate step but one planning and managing a reproductive project from inception to completion. When procreation and child-rearing are carved into a series of isolated acts, the distinction between being married or single, for instance, is irrelevant to the role one is playing in achieving a specific task. A single person or infertile couple may contract with various individuals in securing gametes, embryos or wombs, and it makes no medical difference whether the contracting parties are single or married. Singleness and marriage no longer disclose an ordering of life in which one forecloses the possibility of the other. A single woman forswearing marriage may provide surrogacy services for an infertile couple, while a fertile couple may donate gametes to infertile individuals while forswearing any child-rearing responsibilities. What designates a 'parent' in both instances is the desire to obtain a child.

Although reproductive technology promotes and reinforces the medicalisation of procreation, it is not driven solely by medical considerations. Fertile as well as infertile individuals may employ ART, and quality-control techniques may be used to prevent trivial as well as deleterious characteristics. Furthermore, there is no inherent reason why medical practices employing reproductive technology should ignore or discount traditional marital roles or familial relationships. Is there a larger moral vision driving this emerging pattern?

Procreative liberty

The emerging pattern does not so much reflect a revision of traditional mores governing sexual conduct, procreation and child-rearing as it does a competing account of what gives these activities their meaning and significance. Displacing a normative framework of *marital and familial relationships* in favour of one emphasising *individual interests and rights* entails a collision of contending principles shaping subsequent moral deliberation. Portraying procreation as a series of discrete tasks betrays a substantially differing description of what the birth and the rearing of children encompass, and thereby disparate assessments of what is at stake in employing reproductive technology.

The rudimentary principles of this emerging pattern can be seen in John Robertson's account of *procreative liberty*.[10] According to Robertson, 'procreative liberty is the freedom either to have children or to avoid having them. Although often expressed or realized in the context of a couple, it is first and foremost an individual interest.'[11] Individuals should be free from unwarranted interference in pursuing their reproductive interests, 'because control over whether one reproduces or not is central to personal identity, to dignity, and to the meaning of one's life'.[12] Since most Western societies already protect a married couple's right to reproduce, it may be easily extended to non-married persons, and the use of reproductive technology should 'be accorded the same high protection granted to coital reproduction'.[13]

The single proviso is that the interests of other persons may not be harmed in exercising one's reproductive rights. Thus determining who possesses rights, resolving conflict among contending interests, and what constitutes harm lie at the heart of procreative liberty. Robertson, for instance, admits that establishing the legal status of embryos pits 'deeply felt views about respect for the earliest stages of human life against the needs of infertile couples to create embryos to serve their reproductive goals'.[14] To resolve this conflict, he invokes a developmental framework in which an embryo slowly takes on characteristics resembling those of a person. Allegedly rejecting the extreme options of viewing an embryo as a person or as tissue, an intermediate stance is adopted in which an embryo should be treated with respect because of its potential to become a person, but it is not assigned any formal rights. Since only persons possess rights, they may exercise a right of ownership over their gametes and any embryos they produce, justifying a virtually unrestricted use of reproductive technology.[15]

Employing donated gametes and surrogacy enables *collaborative reproduction*.[16] Such collaboration should not be impeded because there is no empirical evidence that children are harmed in separating biological and social parenthood. The more pressing issue is establishing procedures protecting the interests of *commissioners* (persons seeking assistance) and *collaborators* (donors and surrogates). This protection is provided through preconception contracts that assign commissioners a presumptive status. If collaborators are excluded from child-rearing their role is limited to providing gametes or gestation, while, if included, the duties and limitations of all parties should be specified. If a dispute occurs, the preconception contract trumps 'the claims of donors or surrogates who later insist on a different rearing role than they had agreed upon'.[17] Statutes should define parenthood in contractual terms instead of codifying a biological, genetic or gestational relationship to offspring, ensuring a 'fundamental' right to 'use non-coital means of forming families'.[18] Without these contractual safeguards, infertile couples and individuals without suitable partners are deprived of their right to reproduce, and collaborators are denied opportunities to assist others in achieving their reproductive goals.

Since individuals have a right to seek assistance in pursuing their reproductive interests, Robertson asserts they also have a right to select the characteristics of offspring. Quality control is 'a core part of procreative liberty and should be respected as such. If it is legitimate for parents to want healthy children, then it should be legitimate for them to use both negative and positive techniques to achieve that end.'[19] Selecting the characteristics of offspring may give pregnancy a tentative quality, as well as inspiring prejudicial views of handicapped children and their parents, yet Robertson is confident that adequate safeguards can be instituted.

The reproductive rights of individuals are secure so long as they are free either to ignore or to utilise the results of genetic screening and prenatal testing. Those choosing to ignore test results should be free from pressure by relatives, insurance providers, or government agencies to refrain from reproducing, implant unaffected embryos, or abort affected fetuses. Individuals choosing to act upon such testing, however, have a right to refrain from reproducing, to use unaffected embryos, or to abort undesirable fetuses. A wide range of negative and positive quality-control techniques should be at the disposal of persons attempting to reproduce, for such interventions do not harm offspring but express parental care akin to providing social advantages following birth. If parents may send their children to elite public schools, enrol them in special athletic training programmes, or authorise growth hormone injections, 'why should genetic interventions to enhance normal offspring traits be any less legitimate?'[20]

Robertson asserts that expanded reproductive choice presents no substantial threat to familial relationships. Reproductive technology may actually ease the loneliness of the contemporary world in which preconception contracts promote a spirit of altruistic co-operation. Collaborative reproduction in particular strengthens the family, because 'with its emphasis on enabling a married couple to have and rear biologic offspring, it supports that institution more than it diminishes it, despite the social, psychological, and legal complications that might ensue'.[21] This is especially the case for children because there is no evidence that they are harmed by novel parenting arrangements.

If procreative liberty may serve as the manifesto of this emerging pattern of procreation and child-rearing, then its medicalisation becomes more explicable. Individuals cannot freely pursue their reproductive interests if they are prevented from deploying the requisite techniques in accomplishing the tasks of conception, gestation and child-rearing. They must have a right not to be constrained by such inequalities as infertility, unavailable partners or inferior gametes. The notion of reproductive rights, however, is a theoretical construct, so it would be a mistake to assume that the mere advent of reproductive technology is forcing a sudden reformulation of traditional values. The 'new' that is often affixed to assessments of reproductive technology denotes more a level of technical sophistication than the morality of the goals they are achieving. Previous generations, for example, have approved or repudiated less advanced methods of assisted reproduction such as sexual intercourse with a surrogate, or infanticide as a quality-control technique. There is a more complex relation between the medicalisation of procreation and the theoretical foundations of reproductive rights that we must examine.

Interests, rights and persons

A fundamental tenet of procreative liberty is that individuals have a fundamental right to reproduce, and increasingly they turn to medicine in exercising this right. Medicine is thus displacing marriage as the principal institution ordering procreation, for marital status is irrelevant in pursuing one's reproductive interests. Procreative liberty not only entails this institutional displacement but also requires a corresponding shift in roles and conduct. A medicalised pursuit of procreation does not contain an inherent set of values and virtues but imposes various procedural principles, transforming procreation from something inherently good to a means of self-fulfilment. In short, the medicalisation of procreation is grounded in a theory of social ordering emphasising a free pursuit of one's interests.

Consequently, procreative liberty may be seen as a procedural principle incorporating selective aspects of *modern liberal social theory.* An extensive examination of the principal tenets of modern liberal social theory is beyond the scope this book, but Robert Song offers a concise and illuminating observation. He contends that although there are many differences among liberal theorists there are nonetheless distinctive similarities, such as 'a voluntarist conception of the human subject; a constructivist meta-ethics; an abstract, universalist, and individualist mode of thought; and a broadly progressivist philosophy of history'.[22] If procreative liberty is a procedural application of these larger liberal principles, then it should be possible to identify a contemporary account of medicine from which it derives its rationale. Such a representative account is provided by H. Tristram Engelhardt's depiction of bioethics.[23]

According to Engelhardt, contemporary medicine is practised against the backdrop of a Western philosophical crisis. With the collapse of Christendom and the Enlightenment's failure to fill the void, Western societies lack consensus on a normative practice of medicine. Thus an 'anonymous perspective of reason' is needed in which no religious or moral orthodoxy is imposed or privileged.[24] A secular framework of moral deliberation encompassing a pluralistic world is required, necessitating a neutral mode of public moral discourse.

The role of the moral philosopher in general, and the bioethicist in particular, is not to judge the truth of conflicting claims but to develop credible options among a diverse population. They map the terrain of contending values, identifying procedures for resolving conflict. Engelhardt admits this procedural approach promotes a public life lacking moral depth, but it is the only rational alternative to violent or repressive intolerance. Although a secular bioethic must acknowledge a wide spectrum of moral convictions, freedom is the dominant value, providing negative constraints and positive motivations for harmonising conflicting perspectives. This harmonising effect, however, is drawn in the contradictory directions of autonomy (or permission) and beneficence. What is good can only be willed by autonomous persons, yet one should help others to do what is good. The dilemma is especially pronounced in medicine:

how can beneficent medical care be provided without violating the autonomy of patients?

The solution is to assign these values to separate social domains. Beneficence forms the *content* of private convictions shared by 'friends', whereas autonomy shapes the *procedural* character of public life among 'strangers'.[25] The former is defined in relation to voluntary associations, while the latter governs civil interactions. Autonomy provides an empty public sphere, 'morally committed to *not* being committed to a particular vision of the good', enabling private individuals to pursue 'their own and divergent visions of the good'.[26] Within this empty sphere it can be demonstrated why autonomy must not be violated, but it cannot be shown why beneficence should be compelled. Autonomy trumps beneficence because it is procedures, not normative values, which cut across and consolidate individuals and communities into a peaceful society. *Personhood*, then, plays a pivotal role in setting the boundary between these private and public spheres, because the 'morality of autonomy is the morality of persons'.[27] Consequently, determining who is a person is a crucial issue, and we may gain some insight on how liberal social theorists make this determination by examining the relation between *interests* and *rights*.

Many liberal theorists argue that in order to have a right one must also have a corresponding interest. If there are no interests then no rights can be assigned because they represent claims upon others. Mere existence does not entail inherent interests. A statue, for instance, does not have an interest in being observed, and therefore does not have a right to be displayed in a gallery. Neither does the presence of life bestow any interests or rights. A tree, for example, does not have an interest in remaining intact and therefore a right not to be cut down, nor does a heart have an interest in pumping blood and therefore a right to be spared a high cholesterol diet.

Rights are derived from certain subjective states or qualities. A thing must have an interest in how it is treated in order to have a claim upon others. With respect to humans, only persons have a stake in how they are treated, and therefore only persons have rights. Unlike statues, trees and hearts, persons are interested in how they are treated and have a claim upon others regarding their treatment. Criteria such as sentience, ability to experience pain, conscious awareness, intelligence and rationality have been proposed for defining personhood. Moreover, it is only persons, in virtue of possessing certain interests and rights, who have a moral status. Thus the criteria used to define personhood engender disputes over the moral status of embryos, fetuses and infants.

The principal criterion employed by procreative liberty is *autonomy*. In the absence of consensus over a normative definition of personhood, the ability to assert one's will becomes the overriding consideration in exercising various rights. Only persons who can assert their will to become artists have a right to make statues. Only the owners of a grove have a right to preserve or cut down their trees. Only persons can choose to consume low or high cholesterol diets. It is important to note in each of these instances that the rights in question enable interests willed by persons, and have nothing to do with the status of statues, trees or hearts. These objects cannot assert how they should be treated, and therefore do not possess any interests or rights. It is only persons who can assert how they should be treated and who may exercise those rights enabling a pursuit of their interests.

For procreative liberty, autonomy is the capacity to choose whether one avoids or pursues reproduction. If the latter option is chosen, a person has a right to seek the collaboration of other persons, or control the qualitative outcome of the reproductive process she or he has commissioned. Only commissioners and collaborators have these rights because they are in a position to pursue or assist particular interests. Autonomous personhood is, de facto, the criterion for pursuing these interests and exercising these rights. Embryos and fetuses cannot assert an interest regarding whose gametes should be used in their conception, who provides gestation, whether or not they should be aborted, under what conditions of good or ill health they will be born, or in what social circumstances they will be reared.

Thus neither do they have a right to be protected other than not to be intentionally harmed in ways that would diminish their development as persons following birth.

It may be objected that embryos, fetuses and infants are not routinely treated in such a cavalier manner. Many societies founded upon liberal social and political principles have enacted legal restrictions upon individuals exercising the full range of their reproductive rights, thereby violating their autonomy. In addition, even in more libertarian societies embryos, fetuses and infants are treated, more often than not, as if they are persons. If procreative liberty plays such a central role, how may we account for these discrepancies?

To address this discrepancy, Engelhardt draws a distinction between *strict* and *social* persons.[28] Persons in a strict sense have the ability to assert their will regarding their treatment and desired fate. Only those who are able to choose a particular course of action are persons in a strict sense. Individuals not possessing this requisite autonomy are, strictly speaking, non-persons because they have no will to assert. Embryos and fetuses obviously lack autonomy, leading Engelhardt to contend that they are property and may be used, exchanged or disposed of in accordance with the interests of their owners.

Engelhardt acknowledges that non-persons are often treated as if they are persons, and invokes a notion of social persons to account for this discrepancy. Autonomous persons are free to assign value to various things as objects of their beneficence without implying that the objects have any intrinsic moral status. Persons may display statuary, preserve groves, or consume low cholesterol diets without implying that statues, trees or hearts have objective value. Rather, they are treated with special care because they benefit the interests of the persons assigning them value. In a similar manner, embryos and fetuses may be objects of beneficence. Individuals or societies are free to treat them as if they are persons, but they do so as social persons and not as persons in a strict sense. Thus some societies may impose legislation protecting a wide spectrum of social persons, while others may permit great

latitude in assigning or withholding this status. Yet as Engelhardt contends, the burden rests on justifying constraints
imposed upon the autonomy of persons in a strict sense rather
than protecting the provisional rights of social persons.

The point of this exercise is not to assess the adequacy of
this distinction between strict and social personhood, but to
highlight a central claim of procreative liberty, namely, that the
moral and social ordering of human reproduction is derived
from the assertive will of autonomous persons. The interests
and rights of social persons are secondary considerations, for
they are ultimately objects of a beneficent will.

Given this primacy of the will, procreative liberty also rejects
any claims that rights or moral obligations can be derived from
natural purposes or a normative structure of human relationships. The purpose of a natural process is assigned by persons
in respect to the interests they are pursuing. It cannot be said,
for instance, that since the intrinsic purpose of a statue is to be
observed, or the natural purpose of a grove is to provide wild-
life with a habitat, the former has a right to be displayed and
the latter has a right not to be destroyed. Rather, whatever
purposes and rights statues and groves might be said to have
are assigned by persons in respect to the interests they are
pursuing. The owner of a gallery may give a statue the right
to be displayed for the purpose of increased revenue, or the
owner of a grove may give the trees a right of continuing
existence for the purpose of hunting game. Moreover, these
purposes and rights may be withdrawn in accordance with a
person's changing interests.

A similar argument can be made in regard to human biological processes and organs. Although the purpose of a heart is
to pump blood, it is an instrumental quality enabling a person's
survival. Its purpose of circulating blood does not entitle it to
be treated in ways promoting the efficient performance of its
function. Persons are at liberty to consume high cholesterol
diets if this facilitates a pursuit of interests they value more
highly than good health. A functional purpose presents no

implications outside a biological process or organism because it lays no necessary claim upon the interests of persons.

Likewise, although human embryos and fetuses develop naturally into infants, this does not entitle them to a right to be born. This determination is made by persons in respect to how an embryo or fetus fosters or frustrates a pursuit of their reproductive interests. Any rights embryos or fetuses might enjoy are not the result of an inherent or natural quality, but are assigned by persons in a position to assert their will over their disposition. Objections to reproductive technology on the basis that it distorts natural processes is rejected, because the morality of such intervention is determined by the interests of the persons deploying the techniques.

Nor can rights be derived from so-called normative structures of human relationships. Rather, such relationships enable persons to pursue their interests. It cannot be said that the relationship between artists and their craft confers a right to statues to be displayed, or the relationship between owners and groves prescribes a duty to preserve trees. Artists produce statues in pursuing their artistic interests, while owners of groves may preserve or cut down trees in line with aesthetic or commercial interests. No inherent rights of statues and trees can be derived from these relationships.

Likewise, there is no normative structure regarding the relationship between persons and their bodies. Hearts do not have a right to be spared the ill effects of high cholesterol, nor do persons have a duty to treat their hearts in healthy ways. How persons choose to treat their hearts is determined by the interests they are pursuing. Although it may be in the best interest of many persons to treat their hearts well, this decision is made in respect to certain pursuits being undertaken instead of any normative relationship between persons and their bodies.

A similar pattern holds true regarding the relationship between persons and embryos or fetuses. The fact that persons can create an embryo does not establish a normative relationship between parents and antenatal forms of life. Rather, the creation (or destruction) of embryos is a means of enabling persons to pursue their reproductive interests. Embryos and fetuses do not have a right to life, nor do persons have a duty to allow them to develop fully. Any rights or duties that are assigned or self-imposed reflect the will of those pursuing their reproductive interests.

Consequently, claims that children have a right to be born within a certain type of family, or that parents have a duty to pursue procreation in a prescribed manner, are dismissed as idiosyncratic beliefs that cannot provide a common moral foundation for the social ordering of human reproduction. Although some persons may choose to assign certain rights to antenatal forms of life, or impose certain duties upon themselves, these rights and duties cannot be imposed on others by appealing to a normative parent–child relationship. Again, a society may assign certain rights and duties, but the impetus is that such restrictions promote larger social interests, reflecting the corporate will rather than conforming to a normative structure of familial relationships.

The reason for this extended discussion on interests, rights and autonomous personhood is to demonstrate how procreative liberty is the paradigmatic account of the way in which procreation is coming to be perceived, encapsulating the central tenets of liberal social theory. Procreative liberty is not a radical proposal but provides a representative account of how procreation is now pursued, marking the cultural background against which Christian moral deliberation is conducted. Given its emphasis on the interests and rights of autonomous persons, procreative liberty can accommodate a wide spectrum of moral convictions without resorting to any normative claims concerning the status of antenatal life, natural purposes or structures of human relationships. To enable a pursuit of reproductive interests that is both pluralistic and peaceful, individuals must not impose their normative convictions upon each other, leading to an inevitable 'procedural morality'.[29]

Procreative liberty presupposes a *procedural division* between private and public domains. It is within the private realm of beneficence that individuals identify their reproductive interests, and they pursue these exercising a corresponding set of rights within a public domain that emphasises autonomy. Autonomy, however, is not synonymous with isolation, so agreements must be struck enabling persons to exercise their rights. Consequently, persons should have the right to enter into contracts for the purpose of obtaining children, and medicine plays a crucial role in these agreements in virtue of its ability to deploy the requisite technical means.

Such contractual relationships portray *parenthood as an assertion of the will*. A contract identifies a collaborative course of action in obtaining a child. In this respect, 'parents as commissioners' is an apt image of autonomous persons exercising their reproductive rights. These rights are exercised not only in regard to collaborative relationships, but also over the disposition of property. Gametes, embryos and fetuses may be produced, exchanged and manipulated by persons constructing a family, so that parenthood is a form of ownership. The increasingly central role medicine plays in pursuing procreation cannot be sustained unless the antenatal components are perceived as raw material.

If procreative liberty both reflects and reinforces the emerging pattern of how reproduction and child-rearing are coming to be pursued, then it also shapes the fabric of moral deliberation on reproductive technology. Its stress on the reproductive interests and rights of autonomous persons dictates which questions seize public attention, and what types of moral discourse are permitted in addressing them.

Moreover, the privileged position enjoyed by procreative liberty influences the course of Christian moral deliberation. As will be seen in subsequent chapters, its influence is exerted in one of two ways: either Christian normative claims are prevented from being asserted in the public domain; or the character of Christian moral deliberation on reproductive technology is distorted or diluted. Before examining these issues, however, we must first enquire into why procreative liberty fails to provide an adequate foundation for moral deliberation,

and examine some alternative theological themes for offering a
more adequate foundation.

• •

*Tom and Jane have been married for eight years, and want to start a
family. Unfortunately, Jane has recently undergone surgery that prevents her from producing eggs or becoming pregnant. They are
heartbroken at the prospect of remaining childless, but are reluctant
to adopt a child because they believe that some type of 'natural
connection' with at least one of them is preferable.*

*Jane's unmarried sister, Alice, has offered to act as a surrogate.
Alice will be artificially inseminated with Tom's sperm. Alice will
receive no payment other than reimbursement for medically related
expenses associated with the pregnancy and delivery. Following birth,
she will surrender custody of the child to Tom as the 'natural' father
and Jane as his wife. Should Tom and Jane accept this offer? Why or
why not?*

chapter two

Theological Themes

This chapter provides a theological foundation for the alternative moral framework of procreative stewardship. The first section contends that life is a gift given by God. Since humans belong to God, they should not treat themselves or others as possessions or property. The following section argues against a dualistic understanding of persons in favour of humans as embodied souls and ensouled bodies. The next section claims that marriage provides a normative foundation for a familial covenant of mutual love and fidelity that is uniquely well suited for the procreation and rearing of children. The final section presents the basic tenets of procreative stewardship that will be more fully developed in subsequent chapters.

IN THE PREVIOUS CHAPTER I claimed that procreative liberty provides an inadequate foundation for moral deliberation on reproductive technology. This chapter provides the principal rudiments of an alternative foundation by examining four theological themes.

God's creatures

Following Karl Barth, our lives are not our own. Rather, our lives belong to God and we are each entrusted with a *gift* and *loan* of life.[1] This is not a gift and loan, however, to do with as we please. Since our lives belong to God, there are certain limits and expectations accompanying the gift and loan of life, and humans are accountable for using it properly. Thus we are called to exercise a *stewardship* of the gift and loan that God has entrusted to our care. As stewards of life we do not possess our own lives or those of others, nor may we treat others or ourselves as property.

We receive the gift and loan of life, and exercise our steward-ship of it, as God's *creatures*. Moreover, humans are created in God's image and likeness. To invoke the imagery of Genesis, we are animate dust.[2] This does not suggest that humans are merely fortunate animals who have benefited from certain evolutionary advantages. It implies instead that humans are creatures that God has called to accomplish certain purposes he commands them to accomplish, and in obeying these com-mands they become the kind of creatures God intends them to be. Our lives, as creatures, are not what we will them to be, but involve aligning our wills in conformity with divine expectations.

We may speak, then, about a nature and structure of crea-turely life, especially in respect to our life together with other creatures bearing God's image and likeness. Although we belong to God, we also belong with other creatures. Again following Barth, since our lives are not our own, we can only find true freedom (i.e. what God intends us to be) in obedience to God's commands. Consequently, humans are oriented toward God's service and praise, and drawn to the One who has entrusted them with the gift and loan of life. Yet we do not discover genuine freedom as autonomous individuals, but only in fellowship with others. We are drawn naturally to other creatures bearing God's image and likeness that have also been entrusted with the gift and loan of life.[3]

Yet for what purpose, or to what end, has God created humans? And what is God calling and enabling humans to be and to do in accomplishing this end or purpose? A succinct answer is suggested by God's commanding humans to exercise dominion over creation.[4] Humans are the creatures God has called to govern or order creation in accordance with its creator's intentions. There are three general precepts that may be derived from, as well as help clarify, the meaning of this divine command.

First, *dominion is a blessing*. The charge to govern creation is neither a crushing burden nor an insufferable challenge, testing humans to determine if they are worthy of bearing God's image. Dominion enables humans to become what God intends them to be, namely, the creatures he has authorised to tend what he has created. If humans refuse or neglect this blessing they reject their own nature, as well as the One whose likeness they exhibit. This does not imply that exercising this divine commission is free of demanding responsibilities, but that our labours are inspired by gratitude at being entrusted by God to perform a role reserved only for creatures embodying God's image.

Since dominion is a divine blessing, God expects its recipients to exercise it in accordance with creation's *vindicated order and appointed end in Christ*. According to Oliver O'Donovan, the death, resurrection and ascension of Jesus Christ vindicates creation and its order.[5] The word 'creation' implies a given order; otherwise the universe would consist of undifferentiated matter and energy. Since God's created order includes all creatures and the natural processes upon which they depend, creation's vindication provides an objective and expansive focal point for moral deliberation. This does not mean that we may simply look to nature and discover given norms or ethical principles. This would reduce creation to nature, diminishing the significance of Christ's resurrection. Rather, a vindicated creation discloses a *natural ethic* that can only be perceived in its ordering in and to Christ as the head of creation and firstborn from the dead. It is what Christ's resurrection reveals that enables us to see a created order instead of a more narrowly construed natural order.

Humans, however, cannot simply perceive a created order, for their perception is distorted by what classic theology described as the fall. Humans exhibit a 'fateful leaning towards death' or inclination to 'uncreate' themselves and the 'rest of creation'. In Christ's resurrection, creation and its ordering towards life is vindicated in that humans have 'not been allowed to uncreate what God has created'.[6] Humans are the designated caretakers of creation, possessing the ability to discern God's commands and capacity to execute them at God's bidding. As stewards, humans are authorised to govern creation in accordance with its vindication and re-creation in Christ.

Consequently, humans must act in exercising their dominion and stewardship, performing tasks that are inherent in their role as God's creatures. There is, for instance, the task of *co-operation*. Humans cannot faithfully assert their dominion, or be faithful stewards in isolation from each other. Thus the blessing of dominion is given equally to woman and man; they are commissioned together by God as female and male. Although God's image is fully imprinted upon both, it is not fully expressed in their separation. Their integrity depends upon their fellowship; they are created to be together. They cannot govern creation in accordance with its vindicated order if it is divided between them. Humans cannot receive the blessing of dominion, nor discharge their stewardship, as female or male, but only as women and men in fellowship.

Second, humans are the creatures God has commanded to *subdue the earth*. Although Christ has vindicated creation, it is not yet suitable to be enveloped fully within its appointed destiny. The natural and historical processes enabling creation to be a hospitable habitat for its creatures must be directed in conformity with God's commands and intentions. Subduing the earth may be understood as subjecting it to creation's vindicated order and the lordship of its creator. This requires a delicate balance between asserting and restraining the co-operative powers that God has authorised humans to discharge in exercising their stewardship.

Since humans are commanded by God to subdue the earth, they are also mandated to act in ways directing creation toward its destiny in Christ. Humans are not authorised to recast creation in their own image, or plunder it in satisfying their every want and need. They are not called to vanquish creation but to safeguard it, enabling it to be fully redeemed by God from its futility in the fullness of time. In bearing God's image, humans are called to be trustworthy stewards, subjecting creaturely life to creation's vindicated order, so the imprint of its creator and redeemer becomes more deeply etched upon a work of divine love being drawn toward its consummation.

Humans must acknowledge *God's authority* if they are to accomplish the co-operative tasks God commands them to perform. The world cannot be submitted to creation's vindicated order if there are no creatures authorised by God to act in his behalf. Moreover, if this governance is to be organised properly, there must be sufficient authority to compel requisite acts. The ability to act in a genuinely free and responsible manner requires an acceptance of divinely imposed constraints. These acts must conform to a given pattern and end, for as O'Donovan contends, 'since freedom is not indeterminacy or randomness but purposive action, this means describing the world as a place in which actions may have ends, that is to say, as a teleological system'.[7] Humans, for instance, are not authorised by God to impose their will upon nature as if it were merely raw material. Rather, their acts are limited to directing creation towards its end in Christ. Thus humans are authorised by God to regulate procreation and child-rearing in exercising their dominion and stewardship across generations.

Consequently, humans have been given a mandate to *procreate*. This mandate is, however, proximate instead of ultimate. An orderly transmission of life requires procreative stewardship, enabling humans to complete the tasks God has called and empowered them to accomplish. The command to be fruitful and multiply is not 'pro-natalist' but pro-creative, because it is conducted 'for, or in behalf of (*pro*), the creator of all things'.[8] The dominion and stewardship entrusted to humans places procreation in a normative category beyond, though integrally related to, biological necessity. Humans must organise their reproductive pursuits as a co-operative and divinely appointed task. Sustaining themselves toward an end established by God entails more than passing on genes. It is through their full and complete fellowship as woman and man that offspring are brought into being, and prepared to carry on the co-operative tasks required of their dominion and stewardship.

Embodied creatures

As God's creatures we are also *embodied creatures*. This may appear to be stating the obvious, but given our cultural fascination with asserting the human will over physical limitations, it is worth reminding ourselves that it is through our bodies that we experience our lives as and with other creatures. We are not souls entrapped in bodies, nor bodies that happen to contain souls. Indeed, it is the resurrection of the body, and not the survival of the soul, that is the object of Christian hope. As Augustine makes clear, embodied creatures and not ghostly apparitions will inhabit the New Jerusalem.[9] Consequently, we cannot ignore, manipulate or alter our bodies, or those of others, and then claim these acts do not affect one's soul or shape one's identity. What we do with, through and to our bodies is part of who we are and who we are becoming.

We are living in an era in which the body, both our own and the bodies of others, attracts our attention. We spend an inordinate amount of time, energy and money worrying about, pampering and taking care of our bodies. We are ever searching for novel ways to stimulate or enhance the sensual pleasures our bodies provide us. We are also attracted to the beauty, strength or physical prowess of other bodies, and again spend a great deal of time and money watching the brave and beautiful display their attributes.

The body also repels us. Again, we spend an inordinate amount of time, energy and money attempting to correct or overcome the limitations of our bodies. Through surgery we can sculpt our bodies in a more desirable image and likeness. Through a combination of drugs, medical treatments and sheer will-power we wage a constant war against ageing, attempting to stay young in body as well as heart. We treat any debilitating illness or infirmity as an assault upon our autonomy and mobility, going to great lengths to replace failing organs and preventing the birth of children with deleterious traits to spare them the suffering and indignity of a deteriorating body.

This ambivalence toward the body inspires two attitudes that are pertinent for this discussion: first, there is a tendency to reduce the body to a collection of parts. These parts may, in turn, be manipulated, improved, or even replaced to enhance the life of the person possessing them. In short, we believe that we own our body parts and may do with them largely as we will, albeit within certain practical and legal constraints. This notion of possession, however, reinforces a functional dualism between the body and the mind, will or soul. Altering body parts does not change the essence of one's personhood – grounded in the mind, will or soul – except to the extent that these interventions enable or impede a person in enriching the quality of this essence. Although these reductionistic and dualistic tendencies may promote in many circumstances a more efficient practice of medicine, they nonetheless change our perception of what we are doing and attempting to achieve in manipulating the body parts that we own or acquire. The problem of childlessness, for example, becomes an exercise in correcting or bypassing defective organs or gametes.

Second, this notion of bodily possession intensifies a stronger sense of self-possession; a tendency to believe that we own ourselves. It is through an assertive will that we express who we are, who we want to become, what we wish to achieve. Our relationships, then, are the outcomes of negotiation among self-possessed people. The body does not impose a relational structure among individuals, but is seen as a means or impediment for forming the various bonds of human association that we wilfully pursue.

The imagery of negotiated relationships among self-possessed individuals, however, fails when applied to the parent–child relationship. Children, much less embryos or fetuses, cannot assert who they are, what they want to become or wish to achieve. The relationship between parent and child is not entirely reciprocal, at least in the early stages, so the weaker party may be regarded as a means of satisfying the desires of the stronger party. Yet if this is the case it begs an important question: if children, as well as embryos and fetuses, lack an assertive will and therefore cannot possess themselves, then who does possess them? Despite stringent safeguards, it is difficult to deny that reproductive technology reinforces a perception of parental proprietorship over offspring.

In response to these troubling attitudes, Christians must admit that as God's embodied creatures, humans live in a *good but imperfect creation*. It is reported in Genesis that on the seventh day God rested and proclaimed creation to be very good.[10] Yet this good creation does not result in an entirely hospitable world. Following the rebellious events in Eden, such natural events as earthquakes, drought, famine and disease render the human condition fairly miserable, leading Paul to anticipate a day when creation shall be rescued from its futility.[11] How can it be that a good creation is also the source of pain and suffering? This is why 'creation' and 'nature' are not synonymous terms. Although creation is good because of the imprint it bears of its creator, and its created order has been vindicated by Christ's resurrection, its perfection will be accomplished only in Christ in the fullness of time. In the meantime, as Paul reminds us, we, like creation, groan in travail awaiting the salvation of our bodies.

This does not mean, however, that God forbids humans to ease creation's groaning. Indeed, we may talk about God calling humans to pursue acts of healing. The majority of Jesus' miracles as recorded in the gospels involve a restoration of health, and the Bible portrays medicine as a divine blessing, affirming the work of physicians as a noble calling. This commitment to healing bears witness to creation's destiny in Christ in which all that is not well will be made well. Thus there is no contradiction in affirming that creation is good, while refusing to append the same adjective to such natural phenomena as cancer cells or deleterious genes. Moreover, we may say that part of our lives as embodied creatures involve a

parental concern for the health of offspring. Parents who care-
lessly ignore the health of their children are rightfully judged
to be negligent or incompetent. A pressing moral challenge
now facing us is to what extent, given an expanding range of
quality-control techniques at our disposal, may a genuine
parental concern for the health of children be expressed at the
antenatal stage? Or in theological terms, may we use reproductive technology in an attempt to direct this natural process
toward creation's destiny in Christ? And may we employ it
in such a manner that we are able to resist a reductionistic
understanding of the body and sense of parental proprietorship
over children?

In order to address these questions we must first explore the
need for ordering the male–female and parent–child relationships in a manner emphasising the responsibilities accompanying God's gift and loan of life. As noted previously, God
commands humans to pursue those ends or purposes that
enable them to become the kind of people God intends them
to be. The purpose of the relationship between woman and
man, for instance, is to partake of a mutual fellowship reflecting
the nature of the triune God, whose image and likeness they
bear.[12] It is for the sake of this fellowship that God created
humans as female and male, for without this difference there
can be no genuine fellowship, nor could humans pursue those
purposes that God has commanded them to accomplish. If
humans ignore or discount a moral ordering of their relationship as female and male, then neither can they become women
and men in the kind of fellowship intended for them by their
creator. Thus we must also speak about a normative structure
of marital and familial relationships.

Marriage and family

The fellowship between woman and man is drawn toward
marriage, disclosing a mutual and divinely ordained encounter
between female and male. It must be stressed, however, that

not all women and men are called to marry. Some are called to lives of singleness that nevertheless honour the fellowship of woman and man. In being drawn toward each other as women and men, it is the one-flesh unity of marriage that expresses the fullest and deepest dimension of their fellowship. We may point to marriage as a sign, covenant and vocation bearing witness to a creation being drawn toward the expansive and enfolding love of its creator and redeemer.

As a *sign*, marriage directs our attention toward a life of mutual belonging and sacrificial fellowship. Marriage is not simply a means of self-fulfilment or of pursuing one's reproductive interests. If this were the case, then marriage would be little more than a cumbersome mechanism of self-gratification and ritualised breeding. Rather, marriage is a relationship greater than the sum of its parts. A marriage is not composed of the parallel 'stories' of a woman and a man. Instead, a marriage unfolds as a singular 'story' of a wife and husband whose bond shapes who they become in their life together. Moreover, it is a bond or story of mutual self-sacrifice. In mutually committing themselves to the welfare of the other, a married couple becomes enveloped into a relationship transcending the fulfilment of their respective self-interests.

Thus we may also speak of marriage as a *covenant*. A covenant entails the ordering of goods that are both internal and external to a relationship, binding its parties together by its imposed terms. In contrast to a contract, the terms of a covenant are not subject to periodic negotiation in response to the desires of the parties. A covenant confirms and embodies the given structure of a particular type of relationship, whereas a contract assists individuals in achieving their respective goals. The former directs the will of those in covenant, while the latter is a means for asserting the will of contracting parties. Following Rodney Clapp, a contractual model portrays marriage as an economic transaction between two autonomous persons, striving for a 'union of interests rather than a union of selves'. Such an arrangement presumes that marriage is defined and structured by the 'wants and needs' of the spouses who are not accountable to any larger 'tradition, community, or institution'. A covenantal model entails a joining of two persons 'unconditionally' committed to each other, and since their covenant is made in the eyes of God they are in turn accountable to the church.[13]

Or as Paul Ramsey contends, marriage is a covenant of mutual love and fidelity binding together the full and embodied being of a particular woman and man.[14] Moreover, their covenant is christologically and teleologically oriented – i.e. a marriage is drawn toward its end in Christ. 'Men and women are created covenant, to covenant, and for covenant. Creation is *toward* the love of Christ.'[15] Thus procreation outside of marriage severs the unitive and procreative dimensions of covenantal love, stripping sexual intercourse of its significance when reduced to either reproduction or gratification. Furthermore, although the marital covenant draws a wife and husband together, it does not collapse in upon itself. In their physical joining spouses imply that their fellowship is open to including children. By its nature marriage is oriented toward becoming a family, for it is a 'covenant whose matter is the giving and the receiving of acts which tend both to unique one-flesh unity between the partners and to the unique one flesh of the child beyond them'.[16] In marriage a woman and man give birth to a child to whom both are related and drawn together in love and fidelity.

In faithfully fulfilling the roles as wife and husband in covenant, we may also speak about marriage as a *vocation*. A vocation marks an obedient response to a particular command of God in which one way of life is followed to the exclusion of other possible ways. A vocation orders one's life within those circumstances where one is called to follow Christ. The particularity of a vocation, however, is not synonymous with receiving private instructions from God. Although how one follows a vocation may contain unique qualities, there is nonetheless continuity over time on how a vocation should be followed. Otherwise we could not discern the difference between an obedient and disobedient response to God's command.

In turn, every vocation encompasses an inherent set of *virtues and practices*. A virtue is a quality denoting the excellence of an object or person. Objects or persons are excellent when they embody or personify the requisite quality for which they are fitted. To designate an object or person as being excellent, we must be able to identify the requisite quality. In respect to conduct, a virtue provides a foundation for habitual behaviour that is recognised as being excellent within a given set of circumstances. A person attains a virtuous status when one's character personifies the requisite quality, and to attain this status one must master a fitting set of practices. For example, within marriage there is the virtue of fidelity which when practised faithfully shapes habitually faithful spouses.

Determining which virtues and how they should be practised, however, is not left to personal judgement, but is imposed by the purpose or *telos* of a particular vocation. Every vocation is composed of a teleological ordering of its virtues and practices. Over time, a normative pattern of how these virtues should be practised is established, enabling a vocation to accommodate change while ensuring continuity. For various reasons, how certain virtues are practised may change, enabling a more faithful pursuit of a vocation, yet these changes accord with the vocation's *telos*. This does not imply that new virtues may be arbitrarily introduced or established practices altered, for such innovations may distort the integrity of a vocation. Rather, continuity is safeguarded, and change evoked, within the social contexts to which a vocation is related. For instance, a more equitable sharing of household and child-rearing responsibilities between women and men is a change marking a more faithful practice of covenantal fidelity, thereby safeguarding the integrity of marriage. By contrast, practising sexual liaisons with multiple partners is an innovation corrupting the virtue of marital fidelity, distorting the meaning of marriage as a covenant of habitually faithful spouses.

Thus every vocation is embedded within a tradition-bearing community that discerns whether a change in practising a virtue is continuous with the *telos* it is ordered to serve. It is this embedding that safeguards a vocation while also evoking change in its practices. In the absence of such a tradition-bearing community it is doubtful if we could speak meaningfully about vocation, because 'virtues' are used to assert an individual's preferences rather than ordering a normative pattern of conduct. When no longer embedded in appropriate community, a 'vocation' may become perverted into something other than it attests to be, in turn distorting the 'virtues' that are being 'practised'. It would seem odd, for example, to speak of a community of violent crime whose members practise the virtues of assault and robbery. Yet in the absence of a tradition-bearing community in which lawful and criminal conduct are not clearly differentiated, it is presumably possible to entertain a vocation of liberating assets in which mastering the practice of inducing terror is recognised as a virtue. A vocation derives its intelligibility from a tradition-bearing community, for it is only in such a setting that a fitting set of virtues may be formed, practised and sustained.

We may say that the family is a community in which certain integral vocations are embedded, and from which they derive their intelligibility. In obedience to God's command, a woman and a man are called to the covenant and vocation of marriage. Their marriage marks a unique unfolding of God's ordering of their lives, yet their mutual commitment to each other is continuous with an established pattern of what it means to be married. If God should call them to become parents, then in obedience they follow the vocation of parenthood. This not only entails changes in their marital fellowship, but also a recognition that their new vocation is built upon, and grows out of, the exclusive co-operation of their marriage. God has not called them as individuals to obtain *any* child, but to receive the one entrusted to their care as wife and husband.

The family encompasses practising an inherent set of marital and parental virtues, in which the latter build upon and become intertwined with the former. A marital covenant provides the foundation for a more expansive *familial* covenant of mutual fidelity. The requisite practising of truth-telling, patience and mutual sacrifice in becoming habitually faithful spouses may be drawn upon in becoming habitually faithful parents. These virtues, however, are not idealistic constructs; they are not practised for the sake of spouses and parents in general, but in terms of a particular spouse and child commanding one's fidelity. Yet neither does this imply that each parent–child relationship has its own unique set of virtues and practices, otherwise we could not discern the difference between fidelity and infidelity. Rather, we see in a particular practising of marital and parental fidelity continuity with a normative ordering of marriage, parenthood and the family. How may we identify the patterns of this normative ordering?

First, we may identify marriage and family as providing a place of *mutual and timely belonging*. By this I mean the ordering of human life prior to creation's consummation in Christ. It emphasises the incomplete quality of creaturely life, juxtaposed by the imposed relationships shaping its temporal ordering. In their life together a family situates its members within the temporal unfolding of God's creation. In short, a family is a human association ordained by God in which parents and children belong with each other.

In providing a place of mutual and timely belonging, however, a family is not a theoretical concept, but a covenant of particular individuals bound together under circumstances often not of their choosing, and enduring independently of what they might will or want. This woman belongs with this man in marriage; this child belongs with these parents in this family. A particular person is (or was) my spouse, parent, child or sibling, and this fact cannot be erased through sheer force of will. Although a woman and man may choose to marry each other, with parenthood they become mutually related with someone they did not choose, and who has not chosen them. Yet together they share a unique relatedness unlike any other they may choose to share with others. As their familial relationship unfolds, they come to know themselves and each other as spouse, parent, child and sibling. The nature of this familial covenant requires an enduring fidelity among persons related by both voluntary and involuntary bonds, and faithfully performing one's role within this relationship requires the imposed virtues and practices of their covenant.

Second, marriage and family is a sphere of an *expansive, unfolding and enfolding love.* When God calls a woman and man to marriage, a new and more expansive love unfolds in their exclusive affection and mutual devotion. Their one-flesh unity is the embodiment of their fully shared being. If they become parents, a further unfolding of their love occurs in extending their fellowship to children. The two become one and bring into being a new life. There is, however, a continuity of love originating in marriage and extending through the begetting and rearing of children. The birth of a child does not simply entail the creation of a parallel relationship; a family is not merely a container for its separate spousal, parental, filial and fraternal relationships. Rather, they are related aspects of a larger loyalty, mutual belonging and common love. There is an unfolding of marital love into parental love, and a consequent unfolding of familial love enlarging, enfolding and transforming the forms of love preceding it. Although the family includes marriage, procreation and parenthood, they are not its sum total, nor can it be reduced to any one of these elements. Marriage is the normative foundation of the family because it most clearly embodies the biological and social contours of the relationships that offer a mutual and timely place of belonging.

Familial love, however, is not merely affection or sentiment. It is an outgrowth of following those vocations, and practising those virtues, that are inherent to familial affinity. A family is a community incorporating its members into a common life, but not as a collective diminishing the individual, nor as a contract enabling individuals to pursue their respective interests. Within a familial relationship there is an ordering of individual goods with a common good. Consequently, familial relationships are neither a series of negotiated quid pro quo arrangements, but involve the giving and receiving of loving commands for the sake of the individuals and relationships comprising it. A daughter, for instance, may command her father to fulfil responsibilities incumbent on him as her father not only for her own well-being, but also for the good of their family.

It must be emphasised, however, that although children are properly brought into being through the one-flesh unity of their parents, they are not parental possessions. Rather, children and parents belong together in a family. In a restricted sense there is an adoptive element in every family, for God entrusts children to the care of parents.[17] Parents with children who are not biological offspring constitute an authentic family, so long as a place of mutual and timely belonging is provided. Adoption serves as reminder that although the family consists of a complex nexus of biological and social bonds, it cannot be reduced to either, but requires their suitable ordering, under both ideal and adverse circumstances, so the gift of children may be properly received and nurtured.

Thus we may also speak about the normative structure of the family as a means of safeguarding the nature of procreation. Contrasting 'being' and 'will' is illuminating in this regard. As was seen in the preceding chapter, procreative liberty uses collaborative reproduction and quality control to assert the primacy of the will in pursuing an individual's reproductive interests. Hence John Robertson's emphasis on models of contractual relationships and economic exchange in his portrayal of procreation and child-rearing. Robertson defines parents as 'commissioners' entering into contracts with 'collaborators' providing gametes, embryos or gestation. Moreover, contracts trump any other claim to parentage, for commissioners are the true parents because 'they were the prime movers in bringing all the parties together to produce the child'.[18] Parents are, in short, individuals asserting their will to obtain a child. Although Robertson's emphasis on the reproductive interests and rights of autonomous persons has merit, as Gilbert Meilaender contends: 'When we think of human beings chiefly as "will," as beings characterised by their interests, we see something true, but we miss much else.'[19]

One of the things we miss is the nature or structure of the

parent–child relationship. It is not a relationship among con-
senting parties, nor is it the acquisition of a commissioned
artefact. If it were the former, then ideal offspring would
somehow be autonomous beings who have freely consented to
be children, and if the latter, children would be objects owned
by their commissioners. The parent–child relationship is a
unique bond of radical equality and mutual belonging that
exists independently of the will of the parties.

This is why O'Donovan insists that children should be
begotten instead of *made*. By way of analogy, O'Donovan draws
upon the relationship between the first and second persons of
the Trinity. Unlike creation, the Son is not made but begotten
of the Father; they share a common being. Although we may
say that the Father is the maker of heaven and earth, we may not
say that he is the maker of Christ, the Son of God. Moreover,
making expresses God's will, whereas begetting emphasises
divine being. Creativity based on the will results in making an
object that is unlike and alienated from its maker, whereas what
is begotten is like oneself, sharing a common being.[20]

O'Donovan worries that in a culture already obsessed with
technological and instrumental ways of thinking, we may be
tempted to emulate the wrong form of divine creativity, i.e. we
may come to emphasise parental will over being. When the will
is given priority, procreation becomes a reproductive project
in which the finished product is alienated from its maker. A
fundamental alienation and unfamiliarity is presupposed in
the parent–child relationship. Procreation as an expression of a
common nature, experience and destiny between the shared
being of parent and child becomes displaced by a reproductive
project in which a child is produced as an artefact of parental
will. When being is stressed, procreation is an act of begetting
another with whom one shares a fundamental equality.

Although O'Donovan does not specify when we succumb to
emphasising parental will over being, his point is nonetheless
salutary in reminding us that efforts to produce a child of
one's own may cross a line, becoming indistinguishable from
obtaining a child one owns. Although attempting to determine

when (or if) we transgress this line through particular applications of reproductive technology is beyond the scope of this
chapter, we may, however, devise a moral framework to plot
some points along which such a line could be drawn.

The basic tenets of procreative stewardship

Procreative stewardship is based on a general precept that the
*means employed in ordering procreation should accord with and
enable a more expansive familial love*. This precept is derived from
the family as a covenantal community that is uniquely
equipped to organise a series of co-operative tasks, especially
in respect to procreation and child-rearing. Procreative stewardship necessitates moral deliberation on the extent to which
various technologies may be used to prevent, assist or control
procreation. This section outlines the basic elements of procreative stewardship in contrast to the basic tenets of
procreative liberty.

Procreative stewardship acknowledges that *sexual intercourse
is naturally oriented towards procreation*. This is a condition that
cannot be ignored or discounted. Regardless of how
infrequently conception or pregnancies occur, sexual intercourse is the natural means of bringing a new human life into
being. To the extent that biological processes or organs may be
said to have purposes, we may say that coitus has a reproductive purpose. Proponents of contraception imply that
pregnancy occurs with sufficient regularity to warrant interventions inducing infertility. As will be seen in Chapter 4,
defenders of *Humanae Vitae* are correct in contending that contraception prevents sexual intercourse from accomplishing its
natural purpose. Yet the 'purpose' invoked entails more than a
physical act, for conjugal love is not synonymous with breeding.
Responding faithfully to a parental calling requires that sexual
intercourse embodies certain virtues and practices that are both
related to and transcend its reproductive orientation. Its

purpose is fully disclosed within the moral contexts of marriage and family that are both social and natural in character.

In acknowledging the reproductive orientation of sexual intercourse, procreative stewardship endeavours to safeguard the nature of procreation rather than natural reproduction. The physical joining of a wife and husband is the means God has provided for creating a new human life. Their union embodies the full breadth and depth of their mutual being, so that sexual intercourse signifies an unfolding conjugal love into a larger parental and familial love. The unfolding of this more expansive love, however, does not imply that a couple should produce as many offspring as possible. Rather, it involves a purposeful timing of birth, taking into account the well-being of spouses, parents and children, as well as the good of the family. The reproductive orientation of sexual intercourse is ordered to a larger range of ends that neither trivialise nor embellish its natural purpose.

While acknowledging a natural orientation toward procreation, procreative stewardship also entails an *ordering of sexual intercourse enabling a pursuit of ends that disclose the full breadth and depth of its purposes*. The debate over contraception too often becomes fixated on whether a natural or artificial method of preventing conception best facilitates the personal fulfilment of a couple. Although there is nothing wrong with marriage and parenthood enabling personal fulfilment, the presumption that such fulfilment is an end in itself is troubling. One consequence is that the family is often reduced to a means of self-fulfilment instead of an end ordering how procreation should be pursued. Little attention is directed toward how pursuing procreation may enable or disable a sense of *familial fulfilment*.

Natural or artificial methods of preventing conception may be employed if the purpose is to enable the unfolding of familial love. The intention is not to impede procreation as a means of self-fulfilment, but to prevent an untimely birth. Using contraception in equipping a timely unfolding of familial love is a responsible act, because 'the husband and wife clearly do not tear their own one-flesh unity completely away from all positive response and obedience to the mystery of procreation – a power by which at a later time their own union originates the one flesh of a child'.[21] So long as the reproductive orientation of sexual intercourse is ordered to a timely unfolding of familial love, contraception may also be construed as safeguarding the nature of procreation.

Since sexual intercourse is oriented toward procreation, and its ordering should enable a pursuit of ends disclosing the breadth and depth of its purposes, then the *normative means of procreation is embodied in character*. The physical union of a couple signifies a joining of their entire being from which a new life is brought into being. A child is not the outcome of a reproductive project, but exhibits an unfolding familial love. Thus a child is not a means of self-fulfilment, but the impetus of an expansive and loving fellowship.

It should not be assumed, however, that the embodied character of procreation excludes any technological assistance or intervention. If procreative stewardship allows a proper employment of contraception in ordering fertility, then techniques may also be deployed in ordering infertility. The issue is not technology per se, but how the nature of procreation informs moral deliberation on the extent to which it may be used in assisting an unfolding familial love. Is there a practical standard that may guide such deliberation in respect to specific interventions? The exclusivity of conjugal intimacy is suggestive, for potential interventions may be assessed in regard to how they impinge upon the natural and normative structure of procreation. We may enquire into a range of interventions to determine if a point is reached where the embodied and exclusive character of conjugal intimacy becomes so compromised that it insufficiently resembles an act of exclusive co-operation between a couple.

There is little difficulty justifying drugs or procedures augmenting female or male fertility, provided such treatments are safe, and any potential for multiple conceptions is known in advance. Such measures improve the chances of sexual intercourse accomplishing its natural orientation, and there is no impact on the embodied and exclusive character of conjugal intimacy other than administering diagnostic and therapeutic treatments. Admittedly AIH displaces sexual intercourse, yet conception occurs within the wife's body. Although this technique impinges upon the embodied structure of conjugal intimacy, it nonetheless preserves the exclusive character of spousal co-operation.

It is with IVF that a significant threshold is reached. All that remains of the embodied structure of procreation is gestation and birth, and spousal co-operation has been augmented extensively by medical personnel involved in collecting gametes, fertilisation, and implanting embryos. Does IVF per se, however, distort conjugal intimacy and the embodied character of procreation to such an extent that it is incompatible with an unfolding familial love? Not necessarily. The wife's gestation of a child conceived artificially from her egg and her husband's sperm may sufficiently preserve their conjugal intimacy, as well as the embodied character of procreation, albeit in a diminished manner. With IVF, however, we draw close to a boundary. Even though conjugal co-operation and the embodied character of procreation are preserved, the process begins to resemble a reproductive project instead of assisting the begetting of a child. Care should be taken to ensure that IVF is not used in a desperate attempt to obtain a child. If technology per se does not demarcate a line violating the nature of procreation, then we must enquire further.

Since procreative stewardship acknowledges that sexual intercourse is oriented towards procreation, that its pursuit should disclose the full breadth and depth of its purposes, and that the normative structure of procreation is embodied in character, then *techniques should not be employed which confuse, impede or prevent a clear differentiation of familial roles and relationships*. AID, IVF utilising donated gametes, embryo donation and surrogacy are illustrative points along a line that if transgressed tends to transform procreation into a reproductive project. Although some of these techniques preserve conception or gestation within the wife's body, using donated gametes or embryos entails multiple parentage, not only disfiguring the exclusive nature of spousal co-operation but also distorting parental and filial relationships. A couple, so to speak, reach beyond themselves in securing the biological resources they lack, destroying the symmetry of familial relationships.

Surrogacy is objectionable because gestation, as well as conception in some cases, occurs within a woman's body other than the wife's, disrupting the exclusive nature of spousal co-operation and incorporating multiple parentage. Surrogacy amplifies the more troubling aspects of gamete or embryo donation in disordering familial roles and relationships. This is illustrated in what may be characterised as the 'reproductive direction' surrogacy inspires. The husband (if AI is used) or couple (if IVF is used) go beyond their marriage in collaborating with a woman in obtaining a child to bring back to their family. To a greater extent than gamete or embryo donors, the surrogate signifies a mode of reproduction in which the exclusive nature of conjugal exclusivity and co-operation are ignored.

Employing donated gametes or embryos and surrogacy pay insufficient attention to the symmetrical structure of familial roles and relationships, as well as failing to safeguard the embodied character of procreation. Consequently, these applications of reproductive technology transform the purposes of procreation, how it should be pursued, and what virtues and practices are entailed in that pursuit, transmuting procreation from an embodied manifestation of an unfolding familial love to a reproductive project of satisfying parental desires. The issue at hand is not what is desired, but how and for what purpose it is desired. There is nothing wrong with a couple wanting a child. Their desire to become parents, however, should be fashioned in accordance with the embodied character of procreation and the normative structure of an unfolding familial love. It is one thing to use ART to assist begetting a child and quite another matter to make one. To use a crude analogy, there is nothing wrong with a student wanting an advanced degree. Yet if the student employs a ghost writer to write the thesis, this discloses a distorted desire for achieving this end, one that is incompatible with a normative structure for achieving the degree. The degree is transformed into a commodity to be purchased rather than a status to be earned through the mastery of prescribed skills and expectations, thereby distorting what it means to be a 'student'. Likewise, what it means to be a 'parent' becomes distorted when offspring are obtained as a means of self-fulfilment rather than an expression of mutual and timely belonging.

One effect of this transformed perspective is seen in attempts by advocates of procreative liberty to justify ART on the basis that it assists infertile couples to have children of 'their own'. Yet given how these various techniques are applied, what does it mean, in terms of consistency, to have a child of one's own? It cannot always mean a genetic connection to at least one partner; otherwise embryo donation would not be used. Nor must it entail some embodied dimension involving conception or gestation; otherwise surrogacy would not be employed. And it may not include any genetic relation or embodied dimension in those rare instances when donated eggs and sperm, IVF and surrogacy are used in combination. For an infertile couple to have a child of 'their own' requires embarking on a reproductive project, entailing collaboration with various intermediaries. A parent, then, is one asserting the will to obtain a child. It is this wilful caricature of parenthood that procreative stewardship strives to prevent, for it is premised on the theological conviction that parents do not have children of their own. Rather, children belong to God who entrusts them to the care of parents. A family is a place of timely belonging where, through a covenant of mutual love and fidelity, parents are prepared to receive the gift of children. In short, safeguarding the nature of procreation and familial relationships has more to do with the proper means of receiving children than the goal of producing offspring.

It may be objected that the line drawn in this account of procreative stewardship has been placed either too far or not far enough. On the one hand, allowing contraception, AIH and

IVF (using spouses' gametes) introduces a synthetic element, adulterating procreation from a natural and exclusive act of conjugal co-operation to wilful manipulation. In separating sexual intercourse from fecundity and assisting conception without coitus, inadequate attention is paid to the embodied character of procreation. This leads to the objection, often propounded by some Roman Catholic moral theologians, that the nature of procreation is not sufficiently safeguarded.

On the other hand, prohibiting gamete donation and surrogacy places unwarranted constraints on fulfilling the legitimate desires of infertile couples. The case against non-coital reproduction is symbolic rather than substantive. A couple may use reproductive technology as effectively as their bodies in preparing themselves to receive the gift of a child. Moreover, insisting that a symmetrical structure of familial relationships must be preserved fails to recognise that they are malleable constructs. Employing reproductive technology does not disable the provision of parental care and affection. This leads to two further objections, often offered by some liberal Protestant theologians: that insufficient freedom is granted for establishing families, and that this account of procreative stewardship fails to recognise the social nature of all familial relationships.

These are serious objections and we will address them in the next chapter on childlessness and parenthood. In the following chapters we will also further elaborate the basic elements of procreative stewardship that have been introduced in this chapter.

••

Mary and John are a married couple in their late thirties. For two years they try to start a family, but are unsuccessful. Then it is discovered that John has a very low sperm count. Accordingly, doctors begin acquiring and freezing John's sperm in order to use techniques in conjunction with IVF that will increase the odds of a successful conception. Shortly before Mary's eggs can be obtained

John is killed in an automobile accident. Mary, however, still wants to be a parent and requests that the IVF procedure be performed using the frozen sperm of her dead husband. Should her request be approved or denied? Why?

chapter three

Childlessness and Parenthood

The purpose of this chapter is to explore some possible reasons why people may want to have children. The first section provides an overview of biblical and historical perspectives. The following section examines the extent to which the parent–child relationship is defined by a biological bond. The concluding sections contend that faithfully exercising one's procreative stewardship requires that children should be received as gifts from God that are entrusted into the care of parents.

THE PREVIOUS CHAPTER sketched out a moral framework of procreative stewardship based on the theological themes of life as a gift and loan from God, the embodied character of human life, and the normative structure of marriage and family. It was argued that contraception, AIH and IVF (using spouses' gametes) are permissible interventions in ordering fertility and infertility in accordance with God's commands. The principal objections to this account of procreative stewardship are: it inadequately safeguards the nature of procreation; it grants insufficient freedom in establishing families; and it fails to recognise the social nature of familial relationships.

I address these objections in this chapter by examining why people in general, and Christians in particular, may want to have children. The following section provides an overview of biblical and historical perspectives on marriage, family and singleness within the Christian tradition. The next section explores the issue of the extent to which a parent–child relationship is defined by a biological bond. The final section contends that although a biological bond is a significant element in this relationship, it is not the overriding consideration.

Biblical and historical views

In the Old Testament, children were often seen as a blessing while infertility was viewed as a curse. An individual's social status and role was largely determined through association with a family or household. Moreover, a sense of personal and corporate identity was established and passed on through a lineage. Procreation was understood as both a religious and civic duty, and a family without offspring endured guilt and shame, as well as facing a bleak future. Consequently, it was largely presumed that it was God who opened or closed a womb as a sign of divine judgement or favour.[1]

Early Christian literature on marriage and family must be seen against the religious, social and political backgrounds that helped produce it. According to Santiago Guijarro, 'the family was the central institution of the Mediterranean society of the first century. Through the family, the wealth and social status were transmitted; the individual found support, solidarity and the protection that the state could not give.'[2] Land was the principal source of wealth and prestige. Thus heredity was crucial for maintaining a family's economic well-being over time, and its social status was defined largely in terms of 'genealogy and property'.[3] Although the size and living arrangements of elite and free households varied, a family was usually composed of a father, mother, dependent children, one or more married sons with their wives and children, other family members, and servants and slaves.[4] In addition, the Jewish family served as a primary institution shaping and preserving a sense of religious and ethnic identity. 'The family constituted the key arena for socialisation of each new generation, who would be equipped to raise the following generation, in turn, as Jews.'[5]

For Roman families the principal task was not to preserve a religious and ethnic identity, but to perpetuate a social and political order. The family or *familia* was the heart of pagan society ensuring social and political stability, for the mastery of household virtues was seen as a prerequisite for practising civic virtues. Moreover, the human body was seen as a public resource enabling Rome's survival. The taxation policies of Augustus, for instance, penalised bachelors while rewarding families producing offspring.[6] Reflecting the belief that virtually every aspect of civilisation depended on strong households, Roman citizens were expected 'to expend a requisite proportion of their energy begetting and rearing legitimate children to replace the dead'.[7] As the institution responsible for ordering procreation and child-rearing, the *familia* was a crucial vehicle in fashioning Rome's destiny.

Jesus' teaching against the family must be understood in light of these religious, social and political expectations. Jesus does not denounce the family per se, but condemns familial bonds that supplant a supreme loyalty to God. Jesus commends marriage,[8] and his love of children presumably conveys a blessing on the work of parents.[9] The object of one's highest devotion, however, is not the household, nor does one's hope rest in perpetuating a lineage. Rather, it is out from all partial loyalties that God is calling together the subjects of a universal and eternal kingdom. Family ties are condemned only when they prevent this more expansive allegiance. What Jesus rejects is any notion of salvation through procreation or lineage, for it is spirit rather than blood that will inherit God's kingdom. There is an inevitable tension between familial bonds and bearing witness to God's kingdom.

This tension helps to account for the New Testament's ambivalence toward marriage and the family.[10] Although Christian beliefs challenged familial identity, as seen in a preference for singleness, Christian congregations worshipped within households, inspiring a familial ethos. On the one hand, Christianity 'could not function as an ethnic tradition rooted in the patterns of family life', for conversion entailed a rupture of 'ancestral customs'.[11] As mixed marriages indicate, believers were not required to form new families as an expression of their Christian faith. 'Thus the practical effect of the early Christian movement was not to solidify but to undermine family loyalties for a significant proportion of its adherents.'[12] On the other hand, neither could the church alone provide an adequate alternative ethos for passing on the faith from one generation to the next. Since early Christian communities were often associated with households, a countervailing imagery to anti-family sentiments was offered, providing the rationale for the New Testament's household codes.

This tension between family and church helped shape the life of early Christians. Paul, for example, recognised that maintaining households distracted believers from serving Christ with single-minded devotion. Hence his preference for singleness, and his imagery of the church as the adoptive family of God. Given his expectation of Christ's imminent return, Paul created the greatest possible tension between family and church by emphasising the latter's witness to the end of the present age. Since all temporal institutions were of little significance, given their impending demise, marriage and family could be accommodated without granting them any lasting value. Paul tried to direct the loyalty of believers exclusively to Christ and away from worldly concerns. Yet Paul did not advocate abolishing marriage and family. He counselled believers to remain married to unbelieving spouses, and conceded that it was better to marry than to burn.[13] Rather, the equality of what Stephen Barton describes as the sacred space and time of the church was imparted to the secular space and time of the household.[14] The transformed relationship between Jew and Greek, male and female, master and slave 'radiated outward from the gathered *ecclesia* and into both the broader public life and private homes of Christians'.[15]

Since the stability of Rome drew upon strong households, family loyalty was also an implicit declaration of allegiance to Caesar. Given Rome's pagan religious foundation, familial fidelity was incompatible with the Christian creed that only Jesus is Lord. Paul strove to protect Christians from persecution by counselling an outward conformity to the patriarchal roles of the Roman household, while at the same time subverting them by teaching a radical equality in Christ. Christian households must bear witness to Christ's sovereignty despite their apparent conformity to prevalent social mores. Paul, however, was unable, or perhaps thought it unnecessary, to offer a detailed description of such a household.

This task was undertaken by other Christians as reflected in the household codes.[16] The rapid growth of Christian families required instruction in household governance. Depicting familial roles as ways of serving Christ eased Paul's severe tension, giving marriage and parenthood an inherent value instead of tolerated as encumbrances. The family outlined in these codes is similar to that of a typical Roman household, consisting of a series of relationships between husband and wife, father and child, master and slave. As James Dunn has observed, 'the patriarchal character of the times' is evident in the man asserting his authority over the members of his household.[17] Yet the striking feature of these codes is that, unlike the Roman and Greek models from which they are derived, they are directed to both the weaker and stronger member of each relationship. These household codes attempted to establish marriage and parenthood as valid ways of serving God, not by accommodating prevalent norms but by reconceiving them in terms of a fundamental mutuality and equality in Christ. In short, a family ordered according to Christ provided a witness to the destiny of God's kingdom rather than Caesar's empire.

These household codes, however, were not entirely successful in shaping subsequent Christian teaching on the role of marriage and family within the life of the church. Throughout the patristic period, as Carol Harrison contends, the 'silent majority' of Christians lived in households ordered roughly along the lines summarised above. Yet there was little 'doubt that for most of the Fathers marriage and family life were definitely a second best, preferably to be avoided, and certainly not the place for the leaders, heroes and saints of the church'.[18] Much of the patristic literature contains unfavourable assessments of sexual intercourse, marriage and child-rearing. Although Clement of Alexandria commended marriage as a means of exerting self-control in the 'begetting of children, and in general behaviour',[19] and believed that child-rearing did not distract parents from serving Christ, he was a minority voice among the church Fathers. More typically, marriage was paid cursory lip-service but dismissed as accommodating the worldly desires of half-hearted Christians.

Many of the patristic writers extolled sexual abstinence, often at the expense of procreation. The advantages of virginity were contrasted with the physical rigours of pregnancy, childbirth and running a household, leading frequently to exhaustion, ill health and premature death. This effectively denigrated marriage and parenthood as less than praiseworthy ways of life in comparison to continent singleness where one's time and energy were devoted fully to Christ. Ambrose, for instance, admonished parents to commend holy virginity to their daughters, reminding them that if they were willing to 'entrust their money to man' then how much more honourable it would be to loan their daughters to Christ.[20] Gregory of Nyssa argued that virginity was the only sure road to heaven, because marriage is 'the fire of inevitable pain',[21] and children are doomed to suffer 'so the power of death cannot go on working, if marriage does not supply it with material and prepare victims for this executioner'.[22] Moreover, Tertullian insisted that Christians had no patriotic duty to procreate.[23]

These assessments of marriage and virginity were complicated by a number of ecclesiastical, political and social factors. Established households had become the church's mainstay, raising generations of children within its fold. How could Christian teaching continue to malign this wellspring of the faith by praising a vocation disrupting familial stability? Furthermore, with Christianity emerging as the dominant religion, Christian households took on greater political significance. How was this new prominence to be reconciled with a preference for sexual renunciation? The church was also besieged by various heresies, sharing a belief that the body was evil or polluted, but holding disparate conclusions as to whether this suggested sexual indulgence or abstinence. Yet how could the church teach authoritatively on sexual conduct if the body had little religious significance, as often implied by the patristic writers? In short, the patristic writers had failed to explicate a normative relationship between marriage and singleness.

It is against this background that Augustine established both marriage and virginity as Christian vocations. The task he undertook was not an easy one. On the one hand, he had to portray the value of marriage without challenging the superiority of sexual continence as set forth in Jesus' life and ministry, and Pauline and patristic teaching. On the other hand, he must also affirm the supremacy of virginity without deprecating marriage and family, while at the same time refuting heretical teaching on sexual indulgence or renunciation.

The strategy Augustine employed marked a shift in emphasis on how marriage and virginity were related. Instead of contrasting the latter to the detriment of the former, he compared them as lesser and greater goods. Both were praiseworthy vocations, but one denotes a higher and more difficult way of life than the other. Accordingly, Augustine argued that marriage is the lesser good because it is associated with sexual intercourse and procreation that had become distorted in the fall. Coitus, however, is not inherently evil, nor is procreation a consequence of original sin, for Adam and Eve had been created with bodies designed for begetting offspring. Prior to the fall, Augustine contended, sexual intercourse had been subject to the human will without the disruptive influence of lust. With the fall the bodily means of procreation were now out of control.

Marriage mitigates the fall's disruptive influence by directing lustful desires toward good ends. A woman and man made one in marriage are accompanied by Christ's grace in encountering the necessities of embodied existence. Augustine uses the example of a lame man to illustrate his argument.[24] A lame man attains a good by limping after it. Securing this good is not evil because of the man's disability, but neither is his disability good because he achieves a good end. Likewise marriage, through which the good of procreation is attained, should not be condemned because of lust, but neither is lust good because marriage is good. Rather, marriage 'permits a little limping' in respect to the lust associated with marriage.[25] Sexual limping enables a reordering of life, so the good of marriage may be differentiated from ignominious lust or loss of control.

Augustine's commendation of marriage is based on what has become known as its three goods, namely, *proles*, faith and *sacramentum*. Faith directs lust in assisting a couple to pursue the good of procreation. A faithful couple help restore the rightful place of sexual intercourse in God's created order. Marriage is not a licence for sexual pleasure, but a way of directing human love and anatomy in line with the kind of life God wills for his creatures. Marital fidelity expresses charity (*caritas*) for one's spouse, recognising that lust is part of one's fallen condition, but chastening it to achieve a good end. The sacramental bond carries the greatest weight. Lifelong marriage is inherently, rather than instrumentally, good. A man, for example, may not divorce his infertile wife and marry another woman to pursue the good of offspring.

Since Augustine held marriage in high esteem, why did he continue to insist on the superiority of virginity? With the incarnation the need for procreation decreased while the significance of singleness increased. Before the birth of Jesus procreation was necessary to prepare the time when the Word would be made flesh. Following his birth this purpose was eliminated, elevating virginity as a vocation bearing witness to Christ's return. History is divided into the eras of marriage and continence, and Christians live in the latter rather than the former age. Virginity denotes a higher sanctity. Although marriage is good because it bears witness to God's providential love for creation, it nonetheless retains a compromised relationship with a fallen world. Virginity is greater because it provides a fore-taste, albeit imperfect, of life in Christ's new creation.

To appreciate Augustine's argument, it is crucial to keep in mind that in contrasting marriage and singleness he is not comparing good with bad, but ordering a relationship between ordinary and extraordinary goods. Both are good, but virginity is better in the same way that a mountain is superior to a hill.[26] Marriage and singleness are both Christian vocations, but the former retains a close association with the children of Adam, while the latter enjoys a closer fellowship with the heavenly host of the new Adam. Augustine established a way of per-ceiving these vocations as bearing a distinct, but complementary, witness to creation's redemption, vindication and perfection in Christ. Marriage is oriented to the temporal concerns of the world, affording an ordering of human life in accordance with God's created order. Singleness serves as a reminder that creation is being drawn towards its destiny in Christ. Augustine simultaneously affirms marriage as a provi-dential witness while upholding singleness as an eschatological witness.

More importantly, Augustine set the parameters for sub-sequent deliberation on the moral ordering of procreation. Although marriage and singleness emphasise differing ways of life, together they bear witness to creation's common origin and destiny. The two vocations need each other in bearing a true and complete witness. Thus the necessity for maintaining their distinctive and mutually exclusive virtues and practices.

This Augustinian framework was refined, as well as modi-fied, by subsequent generations of theologians. Thomas Aquinas, for instance, continues to assert the superiority of singleness because it allows one to concentrate on the state of one's soul. Yet he elevates Augustine's understanding of the goods of marriage by insisting that it is both 'an office of nature' and 'a sacrament of the church'.[27] A marriage drawn toward the goods of faith, offspring and sacrament embodies both the natural friendship between women and men, and their fellow-ship in Christ. Marriage does not simply accommodate lust by directing it towards a good end. Rather, sexual desire is inherently good when it manifests a pursuit of the good ends of marriage. Although Thomas does not displace the superiority of singleness, he nonetheless grants a greater parity to marriage by emphasising its intrinsic nobility.

It was with the Reformation that this parity between marriage and singleness was shattered for Protestants. Martin Luther, for example, dismissed celibacy as being unbiblical and unnatural.[28] Marriage and parenthood, however, are honourable vocations, rooted in nature and endorsed by scripture. Although marriage is not a sacrament, it is a divine ordinance that if resisted or ignored leads to fornication and adultery. In the eyes of God there is no superior calling to marriage, and parents exert the greatest form of earthly authority. For Luther, only infertility or sterility excuses a person from this divine ordinance.[29]

In eliminating vocational singleness Protestants placed a heavier burden on the family, for it now had to bear both a providential and eschatological witness. Consequently, subsequent generations of Protestants, especially the Puritans, directed a great deal of attention towards the structure of household governance. Richard Baxter, for instance, argued that a family is a society belonging to God, an instrument of divine providence, a sanctified community and 'baptismal covenant'. In explicating a normative structure of the family, Baxter drew heavily upon the New Testament household codes, focusing on the relationships between husband and wife, parents and children, and masters and servants. In marriage, a woman and man become one flesh who together govern their household and 'help each other in works of charity and hospitality'. The most important household duty, however, was to ensure that children and servants learn and practise the requisite virtues equipping them for some useful role in church or state.[30]

Protestant theologians continued to place additional stress on the significance of marriage and parenthood. In the nineteenth century, for instance, F. D. Maurice contended that the family provided the foundation for a larger social morality. The parent–

child relationship was crucial in learning the principles of a larger and more expansive ethic of universal brotherhood.[31] Horace Bushnell placed even more emphasis on procreation and child-rearing. Believing that both physical and behavioural traits could be passed on and improved from generation to generation, he asserted that God's kingdom would be established on earth through Christians 'outpopulating' inferior races.[32]

There are two items to note regarding this biblical and historical overview. First, Protestants resolved the tension between marriage and singleness by eliminating the vocational status of the latter. As we will see in the next chapter, however, this legacy has prompted some difficult dilemmas regarding a moral assessment of reproductive technology. Second, this heavy emphasis upon the marriage and family begs an important question: to what extent is the parent–child relationship determined by, or limited to, a biological or genetic bond? It is towards addressing this question that we now turn our attention.

A biological structure?

According to Gilbert Meilaender, the moral significance of the biological bond between parent and child is that it serves as a reminder that we are 'embodied creatures who occupy a fixed place in the generations of humankind'. Our lines of 'kinship and descent' shape who we are and situate us within particular relationships and communities, placing necessary limits on our freedom and autonomy. As children and parents, we are bound to people not of our own choosing, learning an important lesson about the given or imposed quality of our lives. Moreover, although the 'sexual union of a man and woman is naturally ordered toward the birth of children', this 'simple biological fact' is not 'governed simply by the rational will'. Rather, a child is a gift of love, a result of a couple's shared being and mutual self-giving. Thus Meilaender concludes that it is 'surely natural for husband and wife to desire a child of "their own" '.[33]

Although there are good reasons for wanting a child of one's own, what measures may be taken to alleviate infertility or childlessness? Are donated gametes, for instance, permissible? If a biological bond is a crucial component of the parent–child relationship, then the answer is apparently no, for the fertile member of a couple and a (usually anonymous) donor would be the 'true' parents. Yet does stressing this biological bond imply that step-parents or adoptive parents are not 'real' parents even though they provide years of loving care and affection? The extent to which biology determines parenthood goes a long way in assessing the morality of various reproductive options as can be seen in the range of representative positions summarised below.

Official Catholic teachings forbid collaborative techniques for two reasons. First, the use of donated gametes or surrogacy violates the one flesh unity of marriage. Although marriage is oriented toward procreation, its unitive dimension becomes distorted when a couple turns to a 'third party' to overcome their infertility. Childless couples are counselled to accept their plight, directing their attention to assisting disadvantaged children through charitable channels. Second, every child has a right to be reared under circumstances incorporating a clear delineation of parentage. Children should not be subjected to an ambiguous parental relationship or uncertain lineage. Consequently, a biological bond is presumably a determinative factor in the parent–child relationship.[34]

Echoing similar themes, Germain Grisez portrays marriage as an open-ended community that is perfected in the birth and rearing of children. It is through their co-operative and self-giving acts as parents that a couple fulfils their marriage.[35] An infertile couple 'can and should try to deal with this condition just as with any other health problem', but this does not include recourse to collaborative or assisted reproductive techniques that would violate the one-flesh unity of their marriage. Rather, such a couple may need to acknowledge that giving birth to offspring is not 'part of their vocation as a married couple', and 'God is calling them to some other form of service to life'. In responding to this calling a couple may still fulfil their marriage through 'true parenthood'. As Grisez contends: 'For parenthood is far more a moral than biological relationship: its essence is not so much in begetting and giving birth as in readiness to accept the gift of life, commitment to nurture it, and faithful fulfillment of that commitment through many years'.[36] Although biology structures a normative pursuit of procreation, it ultimately is not the definitive factor in defining the parent–child relationship.

Although Lisa Sowle Cahill does not condemn ART or collaborative techniques per se, she is nonetheless concerned that such interventions will erode the symmetrical relationship among parents and children. She recommends that non-technological options should be considered. Instead of obtaining a child who is genetically related to only one parent, adoption may prove to be a preferable option for many childless couples.[37] In a similar vein, Christine Gudorf commends sexual intercourse as the preferred reproductive option. Yet neither does she condemn ART or collaborative techniques, given her emphasis on sexual intimacy as a means of mutual pleasure rather than signifying any innate procreative orientation or importance.[38]

Other writers, such as D. Gareth Jones, James Gustafson and Anthony Dyson contend that although a biological bond among parents and offspring is not an insignificant factor, neither is it an overriding concern. Rather, providing a stable environment for rearing children is the principal issue at stake. Such techniques as gamete or embryo donation are permissible so long as the welfare of the child is the primary objective.[39] More radically, Ted Peters insists that a biological bond is irrelevant in expressing a love for children. Thus a wide range of reproductive options and novel 'parenting' situations may express genuine parental love.[40]

This summary discloses that Christians may entertain a wide spectrum of positions on the extent to which a biological bond with offspring defines parenthood, ranging from its absolute necessity to its total irrelevancy. In order to examine this issue of a biological structure of parenthood, we will turn our attention to *adoption* in the following section.

The ends and means of children

Adoption offers an illuminating focal point for our discussion because both opponents and proponents of collaborative reproduction often invoke it. Opponents argue that since an infertile couple may adopt they need not deploy various technologies, whereas proponents may assert that since adoption does not involve any biological bond between parent and child it justifies a virtually unrestricted use of reproductive technologies. Furthermore, examining the following arguments discloses the extent to which procreative liberty informs various portrayals of adoption as a reproductive option.

As mentioned above, Grisez contends that although offspring fulfil a marriage, an infertile couple may nonetheless perfect their relationship through 'true parenthood'. The conspicuous avenue for attaining this perfection is adoption, and it should be pursued analogously to a fertile couple being open to receiving the gift of children. Instead of seeking a so-called desirable child, a couple should adopt a child most in need of care, displaying a readiness to accept whatever child God chooses to give them. This requires a couple to appraise 'their own gifts and limitations', matching them 'with the opportunities for adoption and the needs of babies and children who lack parents'.[41]

Adoption is the only reproductive alternative to coital procreation if an infertile couple are to perfect their marriage through parenthood. Grisez specifies that 'a couple who proceed as they should in identifying the right child will not be daunted by the prospect of adopting a severely handicapped child whom no one else wants and will be open to doing so, unless there are compelling reasons (not emotional motives) excluding that possibility'. Furthermore, he asserts that 'God's grace will enable them to overcome whatever difficulties they encounter in doing his will.'[42]

Although this portrayal of adoption is admirable, it should be noted that Grisez does not indicate what constitutes compelling reasons as opposed to emotional motives, nor does he speculate why God does not equip some natural parents to care for their handicapped children, thereby necessitating adoption. Grisez comes perilously close to implying that it is providential that some parents are unable to care for their children in order that infertile couples may attain higher levels of fulfilment.

In her 'adoption option', Cahill asserts that infertile couples should not restrict themselves to medical treatments but should consider 'nonmedical solutions'.[43] Adoption is such a solution, enabling 'an infertile couple to nurture a child without requiring a reproductive alliance of one member of the couple with a third party'.[44] Cahill commends adoption because it not only maintains a symmetrical relationship among parents and children, but also facilitates a couple to detect 'that other creative ways of satisfying their generative impulses and their desire to share the rewards of childbearing can be found'. Nor is the outlet of these generative impulses limited to adoption, for a couple may respond to their infertility 'through non-parental forms of relationship, service, and fulfillment'.[45] Cahill presumes that in the absence of generative fulfilment some alternative interest may compensate. Thus generative fulfilment is a preponderant motivation rather than a consequence of parenthood.

Moreover, adoption provides a reciprocal relationship between infertile couples and natural parents, converting 'a reproductive "failure" on the one side, and a disrupted birthing situation on the other, into a reconformation [sic] of family relationships. The matching of adults' needs with children's needs is an equation in which a double negative can become a positive accomplishment.'[46] Adoption is a mutually beneficial act, simultaneously alleviating the plight of a childless couple and a parentless child. Consequently, adoption is a preferable reproductive option open to an infertile couple. Cahill differs with Grisez in that, although she holds adoption in high regard, she does not insist that it is the only alternative to natural procreation. Rather, while adoption 'will not be a satisfying solution for all couples experiencing infertility, it is one viable avenue to relieve the suffering that infertility unquestionably brings'.[47] Presumably an infertile couple opts for adoption because of the potential satisfaction it offers.

Peters takes a different tack, insisting that a love for children should be the overriding consideration in choosing a reproductive option. Exhibiting a love for children is unrelated to a genetic connection between parent and child, because their relationship is covenantal rather than biological. There is an 'element of adoption' in 'every adult's relationship to a child, even if the child carries the adult's genes'.[48] Formal adoption is not an anomaly but one option among many that couples may employ in seeking their self-fulfilment. To ensure a love for children, Peters contends that the task 'is to somehow paint responsibility toward others – in this case responsibility toward children – into the self-fulfillment picture. To pull off this trick, I believe, we would need to frame the picture with choice. People will be responsible only if they choose to be responsible.'[49] Since social parentage supersedes any genetic or biological bond, infertile couples may avail themselves of a wide range of reproductive options, including adoption. For Peters, there is little difference in visiting an adoption agency as opposed to a surrogacy broker, for the end result of obtaining a loved child is the same.

It may appear that these authors offer three contending accounts of adoption, yet they share a common presumption that it provides a means of obtaining children for some type of fulfilment. For Grisez, adoption enables an infertile couple to perfect their marriage. For Cahill, child-rearing fulfils a generative impulse in which adoption offers an attractive option in satisfying this aspiration. Whereas for Peters, a love for children is a means of self-fulfilment in which adoption serves as one alternative, among many, for creating a parent–child relationship. Consequently, adoption is portrayed as a reproductive option in each instance, satisfying a parental longing.

Adoption, however, is not a reproductive option, but an act of charity (*caritas*). As O'Donovan argues, adoption sets a 'pattern of representation by replacement' in which 'the social parents of the child act as parents to one who has been begotten by others'.[50] Others assume parental responsibilities in the place of individuals who cannot perform them. Although adoption may enable the marital, generative or self-fulfilment of an infertile couple, it 'retains an element which can only be described adequately as charity – a coming to the aid of natural parents, who have declared that they are unable to discharge their obligations to the child they have brought to life'.[51]

Perceiving adoption as a reproductive option distorts its charitable character, implying a reciprocal exchange or collaboration between natural and adoptive parents. They seemingly enter a joint venture of meeting each other's needs in which the natural parents perform an equally charitable act in surrendering their child to an infertile couple. This portrayal, however, misrepresents the situation as a coincidence of interests rather than a tragedy; i.e. the natural parents' inability to care for their offspring. Suppressing this tragedy opens the door to a market-driven approach to procreation, suggesting that a fertile couple have reproduced for the purpose of supplying an infertile couple with a child. However much adoption may solve the respective problems of infertile and unfortunate couples, to cast it as a reproductive option corrupts the inalienable character of parenthood. In this respect, it must be stressed that natural parents 'do not act for adoptive parents; adoptive parents act for them'.[52] The overriding consideration is the welfare of the child, not the plight of natural or adoptive parents. The intent is not to relieve natural parents of a burden they are unable to bear or to satisfy the parental desires of an infertile couple, but to find a suitable place of timely belonging for a child who would otherwise have none. This is why adoption is not restricted to infertile couples, for its purpose is not to obtain children but to place them in families.

In construing adoption as a reproductive option, each of these authors lends support to John Robertson's attempt at subsuming it into a strategy of collaborative reproduction.[53] If, according to Peters, the primary consideration is a love for children in which genetic relatedness or the embodied character of procreation are irrelevant, then it is not readily apparent why an infertile couple should employ a costly array of reproductive technologies. Presumably, it could be argued, there would be little difference if the less cumbersome method of sexual inter-course were used since the end result would be the same. A fertile wife, for instance, could have sexual intercourse with a 'sperm donor', a fertile husband with a surrogate, or a couple could be contracted to produce and surrender a child for adop-tion. Such arrangements could be justified because they assist the self-fulfilment of the various parties: infertile couples obtain a child to love, while collaborators satisfy altruistic or financial objectives.

In portraying adoption as a way of perfecting marriage, Grisez is in the awkward position of assuming there will always be a plentiful supply of unwanted children, otherwise infertile couples will be deprived of a significant means of fulfilling their marriages. Despite his attempt to claim that marriage is complete in itself – he compares it to a crypt for a great church that was never built, but the crypt retains its inherent integrity as a place of worship[54] – he is hard pressed to console an infertile couple should the supply of adoptive children fall short of demand. His dilemma is caused by maintaining too close a relation between marriage and procreation, for no matter how splendid a crypt may be, it nevertheless stands as a reminder of the intended, but never constructed, church it was meant to serve.

Although Cahill's contention that adoption transforms two negatives into a positive is commendable, it should be a serendi-pitous consequence rather than a motivation. She implies that when natural parents surrender their child for adoption they too are performing an act of charity. If this is the case then perhaps fertile couples should be encouraged to procreate with the intention of surrendering offspring to infertile couples. Yet this would transform adoption into a more altruistic form of surrogacy. In all three instances the principal objection is that children are reduced to some form of personal fulfilment.

Procreative stewardship and receiving the gift of children

With the preceding discussion on adoption in mind, we may now add the final element of procreative stewardship that was sketched out in the previous chapter: *preparation for receiving the gift of children may be either procreative or charitable in character.* Adoption is made a norm by familial belonging while not diminishing the biological structure and normative significance of procreation. An unfolding familial love, based on either a procreative or a charitable foundation, does not alter the natural orientation of sexual intercourse. Rather, it reinforces the need for ordering human fecundity in line with ends manifested in parental and familial forms of love. Moreover, adoption honours the natural orientation of sexual intercourse, for it too discloses the depth and breadth of its inherent and assigned purposes. Adoption is also a way of providing a place of timely belonging within a covenant of mutual fidelity. Nor does adoption contest the embodied character of procreation or biological structure of the parent–child relationship, but provides substitute parental care that has been interrupted. Unlike recourse to techniques employing donated gametes or surrogacy, adoption does not initiate a reproductive project entailing the alienation of parental obligations following birth.

We have now reached a point where the objections to procreative stewardship raised in the previous chapter may be addressed.

First, it was objected that the nature of procreation is inadequately safeguarded. Allowing contraception, AIH and IVF (using spouses' gametes) pays insufficient respect to the embodied character of procreation and exclusivity of spousal co-operation, thereby transforming procreation into a process of manipulation. The strength of this objection lies in what is meant by 'manipulation' and what purposes it serves. It cannot mean intervening in biological processes; otherwise medicine could not be practised. The objection implies that using artificial devices enables a couple to 'cheat' nature in either avoiding or pursuing procreation.

This is a curious objection, for it fails to recognise that any ordering of procreation entails some type of manipulation. Natural birth regulation, for example, involves calculating schedules, as well as monitoring devices in some instances. The dispute, then, is not over manipulation per se, but the extent to which it compromises the biological and normative structures of procreation and parenthood. Making this determination forces the question of purpose: for what end should procreation be pursued? If this question is answered along the lines of some type of fulfilment, then contraception and assisted reproduction may be rejected because they offer an unsatisfying means to achieve a good end. But if the purpose is to enable an unfolding familial love, then there may be good reasons for a limited deployment of techniques to prevent or assist procreation. Noting relevant elements of procreative stewardship examined earlier may highlight some of these reasons.

In ordering human fertility no presumption is made that marriage necessarily connotes a commitment to start a family. God does not call all couples to the vocation of parenthood. However, if God calls a couple to become parents, then the one-flesh unity of marriage is the procreative foundation upon which they prepare themselves to receive the gift of a child. In obedience to God's command, a couple may employ contraception to prevent or regulate the birth of children.

In ordering infertility it must be remembered that AIH or IVF are permitted but not commended. Although the one-flesh unity of marriage is preserved it was conceded that these techniques nonetheless diminish the embodied character of procreation, and the onus is on the couple to discern that they are using these techniques in a manner conforming to the dictates of their procreative stewardship. Indeed, infertility may prompt a couple to consider whether their calling to parenthood should be pursued in a charitable rather than a procreative manner. Admittedly this limited scope of assisted reproduction entails manipulation, but only to a degree that assists an unfolding of familial love. What the objection fails to acknowledge is that some type of manipulative ordering of fertility and infertility is required to evoke a familial bond.

It was also objected that insufficient freedom is permitted for evoking this familial bond. This is demonstrated by the unwarranted significance assigned to the embodied character of procreation and biological structure of parenthood, as well as maintaining a so-called purity of familial relationships. The weight of this objection rests on its understanding of freedom as the absence of external constraints on one's choices. Reproductive technology enhances the freedom of an infertile couple by helping them overcome the limitations of their bodies. Consequently, the symbolic significance of embodied procreation should not prevent them from choosing among a greater range of reproductive options.

In reply, this symbolic significance is also substantive in that it seeks to preserve continuity between procreation and childrearing rather than dividing them into discrete tasks. With the introduction of donated gametes or surrogacy, procreation is changed from an exclusive act of spousal co-operation to a reproductive project. In these instances the technologies employed do not simply compensate what the spouses' bodies lack, but are used to assert their will to obtain a child. The couple commission a project in which the resulting child is the outcome of their disembodied will instead of their embodied being. Insisting that procreation preserve a biological structure of parenthood by retaining the bodily components of the spouses' gametes and maternal gestation serves as a reminder that children are properly begotten from the totality of their parents' shared being rather than made as an artefact of their collaborative will.

Third, to a limited extent the objection that familial

relationships are social rather than biological is correct. The roles of mother, father, child and sibling display a great deal of cultural variability. Yet this is only half the story, for these roles are performed in light of the relation between procreation and child-rearing, and do not simply reflect individual preferences. Disregarding the continuity of these relationships not only undercuts the given quality of familial belonging, but also challenges the rationale of collaborative reproduction. The use of donated gametes and surrogacy is accompanied by a contradiction, for collaborative reproduction is often justified because it enables a couple to have a child they may call 'their own' in a way that does not apply to an adopted child. But if the roles of parent and child are merely social constructs, then it is difficult to imagine how the distinction of what constitutes a child of 'their own' can be maintained, since the relationship is based on what is willed instead of what is imposed. What is being played out is an ideological account of freedom as autonomy in which the family is a contractual arrangement enabling the personal fulfilment of its members, especially the parents.

It is this emphasis upon autonomy that distorts the quality of familial belonging by reducing a child to an outcome of parental will rather than the fruition of a marital bond. In attempting to overcome their bodily limitations, a couple reaches, so to speak, beyond their marriage to obtain the necessary gametes, embryos or womb to establish a parent–child relationship. Consequently, the child is a constant reminder of a missing parent, thereby distorting a symmetrical sense of familial belonging among mother, father and child.

Again it may be objected that there is nothing particularly troubling about a missing parent. Adoptive, blended and single-parent families must deal with this absence, and many do so very well. Although there are similarities, the two situations are not identical. A parent is absent in an adoptive, blended or single-parent family often because of tragic circumstances (e.g. inability to provide childcare, divorce or death) unrelated to the so-called reproductive goals of the rearing parent or parents. It is the step-parent or remaining parent, not the child, who bears the burden or significance of the missing parent. When donated gametes, embryos or surrogacy are used, it is the child who embodies the missing parent.

As has been argued in this chapter, it is understandable that a couple may want offspring and are deeply saddened if they are unable to conceive, bear and raise a child. The suffering caused by childlessness should not be underestimated, and infertile couples are especially in need of the church's support and pastoral care. Yet Christians must also affirm, in Meilaender's words, 'that The Child has come and lived among us and that all who follow him have been joined in one family as brothers and sisters. Without in any way undervaluing the presence of children, we should also be free of the idolatrous desire to have them at any cost – as our project rather than God's gift.'[55]

Consequently, asserting a natural and healthy desire to produce offspring over the limits imposed upon us by our lives as embodied creatures is to transform procreation as a response to God's calling into a wilful reproductive project. And through such projects we may also come to shape ourselves and our children in an image other than the one intended by God. Again as Meilaender reminds us, 'procreation is primarily neither the exercise of a right nor a means of self-fulfillment. It is, by God's blessing, the internal fruition of the act of love, and it is a task undertaken at God's command for the sustaining of human life.'[56]

This chapter has addressed the principal objections to procreative stewardship introduced in the previous chapter by focusing on the biological structure of parenthood and adoption. It was argued that although the biological structure of the parent–child relationship is a significant consideration that cannot be easily ignored or dismissed, it is not the overriding consideration. Parenthood consists of social, biological and normative bonds with children that in turn shape adoption as a substitute provision of care. Thus adoption may be said to honour the nature of procreation and parenthood while not justifying collaborative reproduction. Yet this discussion leaves unanswered an important question: to what extent may humans intervene in natural processes in exercising their procreative stewardship?

....

Peter and Iris are a young couple who have been married for two years. They have been trying to start a family, but unfortunately Iris is unable to conceive a child within her body. They have initiated an IVF process resulting in four embryos when Peter is diagnosed as having an advanced brain cancer. The embryos are frozen following the diagnosis. Despite aggressive treatment, Peter dies a few months later.

Following Peter's death, Iris requests that the frozen embryos be destroyed. Peter's parents, however, produce a letter he wrote to them shortly before his death indicating a strong desire to give his parents a grandchild. Peter's parents request that, since Iris is unwilling to have the embryos implanted in her, they be allowed to find a surrogate in order to fulfil Peter's 'deathbed request'. They have intimated that Peter's sister would be willing to act as a surrogate. Whose request should be granted or denied? Why?

chapter four

Preventing and Assisting Reproduction

This chapter examines the extent to which humans may intervene in natural processes in order either to assist or prevent
procreation. The first two sections review a range of arguments regarding the morality of contraception and assisted
reproduction. The final section examines technology as a
means of enabling or distorting one's procreative stewardship.

IN APRIL 2000, an international research team announced a
breakthrough in infertility treatment that will enable couples
to use donated eggs to produce offspring that are genetically
related to both parents. The procedure involves removing the
nucleus of a donated egg and replacing it with one obtained
from the 'infertile' woman. Using IVF, the reconstructed egg
would be fertilised with her partner's sperm. The technique
will help women whose embryos fail to develop because of
cytoplasmic defects. Cytoplasm is material surrounding the
nucleus, containing a small number of genes. This approach
will allow a couple to use donated eggs to produce offspring
to whom both are genetically related (other than the thirty-
seven extra-nuclear genes contained in the cytoplasm of the
donated egg). To date, no reconstructed egg has been fertilised
or implanted because of 'restrictive' European laws.

On the face of it such a procedure meets the criteria of

procreative stewardship being developed in this book. A donated egg is used to preserve a genetic link to both parents without recourse to a surrogate, suggesting that a restricted element of collaborative reproduction is permissible. However, although such a procedure may honour the technical terms of procreative stewardship, it also seems to challenge its spirit by transforming procreation into a limited, but nonetheless highly sophisticated, reproductive project. As Gilbert Meilaender has written, to 'conceive, bear, give birth to, and rear a child ought to be an affirmation and a recognition: affirmation of the good of life that we ourselves are *given*; recognition that this life bears its *own* creative power to which we should be faithful'.[1]

Meilaender's observation raises two important questions for this theological enquiry into the ethics of reproductive technology. First, to what extent should natural processes inform a moral pursuit of procreation? Second, does the deployment of reproductive technology alter our perception of the principal moral issues at stake in this pursuit?

In addressing these questions, the following two sections review the disputes over contraception inspired by Pope Paul VI's encyclical *Humanae Vitae*, and how these debates influenced subsequent Christian moral arguments on reproductive technology. Using these summaries as a context, the final section examines how reproductive technology may inform, as well as distort, a faithful practising of procreative stewardship.

Preventing reproduction

It may seem odd that a book on the ethics of reproductive technology would devote a section to contraception. Yet, as will be demonstrated, earlier arguments over the morality of regulating human fertility went far in shaping subsequent debates over the ethics of ordering human infertility. What is at stake in many of these disputes is whether the ability to control reproductive processes either enhances or jeopardises human freedom and dignity.

Before the promulgation of *Humanae Vitae* in 1968, there was wide spread anticipation that Roman Catholic prohibitions would be relaxed. Given the development of new techniques, population concerns and reforms of Vatican II, many assumed that Paul VI would position the church's moral teaching in response to the growing need to regulate procreation. The encyclical, however, forbade any method of artificial birth regulation.

According to *Humanae Vitae*, humankind has reached a crucial moment in its evolution, given its expanding capacity to control its propagation. This prospect raises the issue of 'whether, because people are more conscious today of their responsibilities, the time has come when the transmission of life should be regulated by their intelligence and will rather then through the specific rhythms of their own bodies'.[2] A moral response must be based on natural law and divine revelation, for in following their precepts 'married people collaborate freely and responsibly with God the Creator'.[3] Marriage is foundational to the encyclical's argument because it is the normative context governing the transmission of human life. The sacred union of a woman and man, originating in and manifesting God's love, provides the proper environment for the birth and education of children.

Although marriage satisfies many physical and emotional needs, it is not rooted exclusively in nature. A person has the capacity to transcend these needs, giving marriage a deeper character than mutual gratification. Conjugal love does not turn in upon itself, but prompts a couple to extend their fellowship to children. Appealing to Vatican II, *Humanae Vitae* emphasises: 'Marriage and conjugal love are by their nature ordained toward the procreation and education of children. Children are really the supreme gift of marriage and contribute in the highest degree to parents' welfare.'[4]

The encyclical enjoins spouses to exhibit self-control, assessing relevant physical, economic and psychological factors in determining the size of their families. In exercising this responsibility, however, they are not free to use any available means, but may only employ methods corresponding to God's will, following a natural course of ordering the interval between births. Coitus, for instance, is licit during infertile periods, but infertility may not be artificially induced. Sexual intercourse must not be separated from its potential for transmitting life, because marriage is oriented toward fecundity.

Marriage, then, is constituted by its procreative and unitive significance, and violating either aspect impairs it as a way of collaborating with God. The encyclical declares that the 'direct interruption of the generative process', once initiated, is 'absolutely excluded as a lawful means of regulating the number of children'. In short, contraception perverts marriage, for 'it is a serious error to think that a whole married life of otherwise normal relations can justify sexual intercourse which is deliberately contraceptive and so intrinsically wrong'.[5]

Reactions to *Humanae Vitae* inspired a wide-ranging debate, much of it focused on the purpose of sexual intercourse. Defenders of the encyclical claimed that frustrating its procreative purpose diminishes marital fulfilment, whereas critics asserted that spouses must be free to assign either a unitive or a procreative purpose to sexual acts in promoting their mutual fulfilment. For the defenders, marriage orders sexual conduct in conformity to a given natural purpose while, for the critics, sex is primarily a means of enriching interpersonal relationships. Defenders charged critics with subsuming the procreative aspect into the unitive, whereas critics countered that their adversaries relegated the unitive to an inferior status.

A variety of criticisms were lodged against the encyclical. Charles Curran argued that humans achieve their true potential in overcoming capricious natural processes and limitations. Although humans were once forced to accommodate themselves 'to the rhythms of nature', they must now 'interfere with the laws of nature to make human life more human'. Intervening in the reproductive process should be judged in accordance with the humanising purposes for which various techniques are employed.[6] In a similar vein, Karl Rahner questioned if prohibiting contraception prevented couples from collaborating responsibly with God by withholding a reliable method for regulating births.[7]

Bernard Häring contended that exercising dominion over the human body requires controlling biological processes transmitting life.[8] Such intervention is presumed by standard medical treatment in which 'biological functions are often upset' in restoring a person's health, charging the encyclical with subordinating personal welfare to outmoded laws of biology.[9] The most reliable method for exerting dominion over the body is by artificially regulating fertility, and contraception should be assessed in accordance with the well-being of persons exercising this dominion. Richard McCormick echoed similar themes, objecting to the encyclical's teaching that contraception is intrinsically evil because it wilfully prevents conception, imparting a significance that occurs infrequently; i.e. more often than not, sexual intercourse does not produce a fertilised egg. Reproductive decisions should be proportional to the goods a couple is pursuing, so that preventing procreation may in some circumstances be permissible.[10]

Sidney Callahan employed a variety of arguments supporting contraception. First, inducing infertility simulates a natural process since women are sterile throughout much of their lives. Thus controlling fertility 'seems a rational function in subduing nature'. Second, since human nature and historical circumstances are changing, coitus is now oriented toward the unitive rather than procreative aspect of marriage. In an overcrowded world the value of procreation is diminished, so contraception enables greater personal fulfilment while promoting the common good. Third, contraception facilitates better child-rearing. Not only may limited amounts of time, attention and finances be distributed more prudently among a smaller number of offspring, but contraception assists spouses in maintaining an 'erotic tension' helping children to mature properly.[11]

A number of approaches have also been employed defending *Humanae Vitae*. Janet Smith has offered a twofold defence: first, contraception violates natural law because it prevents sexual intercourse from completing its procreative purpose. Acts assisting a biological process or organ to achieve their inherent purposes are, prima facie, good, whereas acts preventing or retarding these proclivities are, prima facie, unnatural breaches of right reason and therefore evil.[12] Second, contraception is wrong on personalist grounds because it diminishes the mutual self-giving nature of marriage. Contrary to critics, who portray the procreative and unitive aspects as contending elements, 'the procreative values of sexuality ... may be vital to the full realization of personalist values'.[13]

According to Germain Grisez, every act of sexual intercourse must retain its potential to transmit life, and deliberately inhibiting this capacity is intrinsically evil or contra-life.[14] In addition, Grisez contends that since the procreative and unitive aspects are integrally related in the one-flesh unity of marriage, contraception distorts this unity, preventing spouses from attaining the mutual and personal fulfilment it affords.

The disputes engendered by *Humanae Vitae* demarcate a fundamental divide regarding the ordering of human fertility. On one side, defenders assert that regulating birth should conform to biological purposes – hence the permissibility of sexual intercourse during naturally infertile periods. On the other side, critics retort that overcoming biological constraints enhances the quality of human life – thus the need for artificially inducing infertility. *Humanae Vitae* sparked a moral and theological debate over whether natural or artificial means for ordering procreation promote higher levels of human fulfilment. Yet how are these positions played out when the issue shifts from preventing to assisting procreation?

Assisting reproduction

Nineteen years after the promulgation of *Humanae Vitae*, the Congregation for the Doctrine of the Faith issued *Donum Vitae* to provide instruction on 'biomedical techniques which make it possible to intervene in the initial phase of the life of a human being and in the very process of procreation and their conformity with the principles of Catholic morality'.[15] Although this document was examined briefly in the previous chapter, a more extensive overview is in order at this juncture.

The issuing of *Donum Vitae* was not prompted by an aversion to medical science, but to ensure that it is employed in ways respecting the 'inalienable rights' of persons 'according to the design and will of God'.[16] Procreation should be pursued in ways acknowledging the spiritual and physical totality of embodied persons, honouring a fundamental right to life and the inherent dignity of all persons. Specifically, reproductive technology should be evaluated by a standard of 'the life of the human being called into existence and the special nature of the transmission of human life in marriage'.[17]

Given these principles, *Donum Vitae* prohibits virtually all artificial techniques assisting human reproduction. The first set of prohibitions focuses on the dignity of embryos, while a second set concentrates on marriage as the normative context of procreation. Since personhood begins at conception, proper respect must be shown to embryos in their creation and development. A new life should only be brought into being through means that respect a person's dignity. Consequently, embryos should not be created for the purpose of improving the chances of pregnancy, nor should disembodied forms of conception be employed. On these grounds IVF, for instance, is wrong because it often involves destroying unneeded embryos, as well as using a non-coital method of conception.

All artificial methods of achieving conception are illicit because they violate the one-flesh unity of marriage that upholds the dignity of both parents and child. *Heterologous* techniques (e.g. donated gametes) are wrong because they divest children of a biological relation to their parents, as well as rupturing the integral social dimensions of parenthood. *Homologous* methods (e.g. AIH) are also wrong because although no donated gametes, embryos or wombs are involved, the techniques disrupt the unitive meaning of marriage.

In two respects *Donum Vitae* builds upon *Humanae Vitae* in condemning assisted reproduction. At one level, it extends the

argument concerning the natural ends and means of procreation. Since it is wrong to prevent conception artificially, so
it is also wrong to assist it artificially. The natural process of
transmitting human life is sacrosanct, and its embodied structure should not be violated. At another level *Donum Vitae* argues
that reproductive technology is wrong because it disrupts the
relation between the unitive and procreative aspects of marriage, thereby diminishing the dignity of spouses and offspring.
This is especially the case with children who have a right to be
born within marriage, and reared by parents to whom they are
genetically related. In this instance, *Donum Vitae* shifts the
debate over contraception away from the purpose of sexual
intercourse, and toward a normative parent–child relationship.

In reaction to these claims, disputants may be placed along
a spectrum on the extent to which they define the purpose of
parenthood as being given or assigned. For those stressing the
former, parenthood is the fruition of marriage. Non-embodied
methods of procreation distort the relation between marriage
and parenthood, depriving spouses and children of their
dignity. Consequently, most reproductive technologies are
inherently wrong. For those emphasising the latter, parenthood
is the outcome of reproductive decisions in response to natural
parental desires. An infertile couple using a non-embodied technique do not necessarily violate the integrity of their marriage,
nor diminish their dignity or that of their children. Reproductive technology should be assessed in terms of the assigned
purposes they are deployed to achieve.

The disputes sparked by *Donum Vitae* have concentrated on
questions of personhood, rights and dignity. For example: are
embryos persons? Do heterologous techniques adversely affect
the rights of children or the dignity of spouses? Does gamete
donation or surrogacy adulterate the integrity of marriage?
How these types of questions are answered has helped shape
disparate moral assessments of reproductive technology, so
Donum Vitae provides a representative baseline for mapping
out a range of positions on ART.

Grisez, for instance, repudiates all forms of assisted

reproduction because it violates the integrity of marriage, as well as the dignity of offspring,[18] while Stanley Hauerwas dismisses techniques such as IVF as unnecessary in practising the parental vocation.[19] Other writers are more concerned that asserting greater control over reproduction distorts the moral and theological significance of parenthood. Oliver O'Donovan, for example, argues that reproductive technology transforms procreation from a good to a project, perverting the nature of parenthood by commodifying children.[20] Thomas Shannon and Lisa Sowle Cahill commend *Donum Vitae* for raising concerns over the potential ill effects on human life in its earliest stages of development.[21]

Another position rejects heterologous techniques while allowing a restricted use of homologous methods. Paul Ramsey approves AIH as a therapeutic treatment, while disapproving IVF because it opens the door to dehumanising experimentation.[22] He also shares the concern that exerting too much control over procreation distorts the normative structure of marriage and parenthood. McCormick, however, asserts that reproductive technology does not necessarily imperil parenthood, provided it enables the birth of a child as the embodiment of conjugal love. Homologous IVF is permissible if embryo wastage is minimised, and abortion is ruled out following implantation.[23] Rahner adopts a similar stance, suggesting that whereas AID disrupts the integrity of marriage, other techniques can be employed in ways that uphold the unitive and procreative aspects of marriage.[24]

A final position contends that reproductive technology presents no ethical problems so long as its use is guided by moral principles respecting the dignity of spouses and children. Callahan, for instance, argues that exerting greater control exhibits a rational human nature, but would restrict access to homologous applications because of adverse effects upon children.[25] Curran is more open to heterologous methods, implying that particular cases must incorporate varying historical and social perspectives.[26] In a similar vein, James Gustafson asserts that policies governing assisted reproduction should strike a balance between individual rights and social benefits.[27] For D. Gareth Jones, assisting reproduction should not prompt any moral objections provided adequate safeguards are followed and children are raised in stable environments,[28] while Ted Peters contends that since biological relatedness is irrelevant in expressing parental love, gamete donation, surrogacy and a range of other techniques may be employed.[29]

As the preceding discussions suggest, *Humanae Vitae* and *Donum Vitae* may serve as landmarks for plotting points within the field of Christian moral deliberation on the ordering of human fertility and infertility. In this respect, disputes over contraception and assisted reproduction are not unrelated issues, but are dimensions of a larger issue on the extent to which humans should control the means and outcomes of their propagation. These documents have helped focus attention on whether nature or the will should dictate the ordering of pro-creation, and whether technological interventions tend to exert a destructive, benign or beneficial influence on this ordering.

It would be mistaken, however, to see these documents as only providing a dividing line and baseline for charting various moral positions. Rather, the positions themselves reflect certain theoretical presuppositions concerning social ordering that in turn shape the mode of moral deliberation employed, and thus which questions are posed, and more importantly, which are excluded.

Most of the moral disputes over assisted or collaborative reproduction have tended to concentrate on reconciling conflicting rights or the extent to which a particular understanding of marriage should shape and limit the pursuit of one's reproductive interests. The right of an embryo to be born or the right of a child to be raised within a particular type of family, for instance, is pitted against the rights of individuals to pursue their reproductive interests. Given the dominant position of procreative liberty, however, normative objections against assisted or collaborative reproduction are rendered mute. Since embryos are not persons they do not have a right to be born, and children do not have a right to be reared by their biological parents since there is no evidence they are harmed in their absence. Moreover, marriage may or may not include certain self-imposed restrictions, depending on how individuals choose to pursue their reproductive interests. Any normative objections (other than harm) are reduced to emotive appeals to pursue one course of action as opposed to another. The very manner in which the principal issues accompanying assisted or collaborative reproduction have been posed and argued betrays the extent to which procreative liberty has shaped the course of Christian moral deliberation.

Rather than arguing on terms dictated by procreative liberty, a more productive approach for Christian ethics is to engage in an alternative criticism of reproductive technology, thereby posing a different set of moral questions and subsequent deliberation. One potentially fruitful path to explore is how reproductive technology itself alters our perception of procreation, and consequently what is at stake in how it is pursued.

Technology and stewardship

One of the most penetrating criticisms of procreative liberty is that it promotes a perception of children as commodities. A virtually unrestricted use of reproductive technology reduces children to artefacts of a 'commissioner's' will. To appreciate the strength of this criticism, we must first examine a critique of technology in general and its distorting influence on contemporary moral deliberation that is often presupposed by these critics. Although an extensive review of these critical assessments is beyond the scope of this chapter, a brief overview of George Grant's account of 'technological neutrality' will suffice.

According to Grant, technology is 'the endeavour which summons forth everything (both human and non-human) to give its reasons, and through the summoning of those reasons turns the world into potential raw material, at the disposal of our "creative" wills'.[30] Such summoning is not a neutral enterprise, for it collapses what were once the distinguishable 'activities of knowing and making' into a singular act.[31] This co-penetration marks a presumably liberating ability to assert the human will over both nature and history, inspiring further inquiry into both in order to master them.

It is important to note that technological artefacts per se are not condemned, but rather the corrupting influence that technology – as a summoning and manipulation of what is summoned – has upon moral deliberation, reducing it to a procedural process of matching solutions with problems. Moreover, what comes to be seen as a problem and its solution are defined largely in terms of technological capability and potential. Thus technology is more than an array of neutral instruments, but serves as a unifying principle pervading virtually every facet of contemporary life.

Portraying technology as a neutral set of instruments is misleading. Such neutrality implies that a technology is not accompanied by an ethic for how it should be used, but is instead assigned by its users. What this portrayal fails to acknowledge is that the very instrumentality of technology imposes its purposes upon the user, for technologies are designed to achieve specific ends which enfold those using them in their destinies. Grant illustrates the effect of a technological destiny by invoking the words of a computer scientist who assures us that the 'computer does not impose on us the ways it should be used'.[32] We are free to use computers in whatever ways we choose. Yet this is clearly not the case, because a computer can only be used within the imposed constraints of its design, requiring that data be abstracted, stored and retrieved in ways explicable to a limited frame of reference. This frame of reference is akin to a 'destiny, without which computers would not exist. And like all destinies, they "impose".'[33] The image of technological neutrality hides its accompanying destiny by reducing freedom to selecting among various options. Technology appears to be an efficient means for people to assert their will over raw material, but it is a form of control limited to arranging blocks rather than exercising an absolute fiat or unlimited creativity.

The most misleading feature of technological neutrality, however, is that such terms as 'person', 'will' and 'freedom' are not impartial descriptions, but normative concepts defined within an unfolding destiny. There is no neutral standpoint to determine who a person is, how the will should be asserted, or what freedom means other than in categories already embedded in a framework of technical efficiency and instrumentality. Technology delivers its purported mastery over natural constraints because it enables a sense of the autonomy, wilfulness and freedom that have come to be expected within a destiny of technique.

Those who presume that technology emancipates people from natural constraints fail to recognise that they become equally constrained by the imposed destiny of technical skill and planning in which they are already enveloped. Moderns deceive themselves into believing that the quality of their freedom is proportional to the quantity of options at their disposal. It is worth quoting Grant at some length in this regard:

> To put the matter crudely: when we represent technology to ourselves through its own common sense we think of ourselves as picking and choosing in a supermarket, rather than within the analogy of a package deal. We have bought a package deal of far more fundamental novelness than simply a set of instruments under our control. It is a destiny that enfolds us in its own conceptions of instrumentality and purposiveness.[34]

There are two important points to note in Grant's observation: first, the process of picking and choosing is itself a package deal. The freedom to choose is exercised only within the parameters of imposed constraints. These constraints constitute the range of choices that may be made, so such normative concepts as autonomy, will and freedom invoked in one's picking and choosing are not external values governing the uses of technology, but derive their intelligibility from within the 'common sense' of the package deal.

Second, the control afforded by technology is illusory. The

'mastery' it offers merely expands a range of available options. It is the chooser, however, who becomes mastered by the options, for persons are reduced to composites of their choices. Moreover, such choosing reflects an impoverished understanding of creativity, because an expanding range of choices does not so much entail the creation of novel values in reaction to technological developments, as it distorts established goods in accommodating a selection process. Consequently, becoming enfolded into a technological destiny requires a fundamental alteration of moral vision. 'The coming to be of technology has required changes in what we think is good, what we think good is, how we conceive sanity and madness, justice and injustice, rationality and irrationality, beauty and ugliness.'[35]

Procreative liberty fails to address this question of destiny, a serious omission since it purports to guide an irresistible 'desire for greater control of the reproductive process'.[36] Yet the 'just' procedures propounded for satisfying this desire never acknowledge how the ensuing reproductive choices initiate the unfolding of a destiny that enfolds the very notion of justice within the imposed constraints of exerting greater control. This omission is especially telling in respect to reproductive technology. Since procreative liberty presumes that an individual's identity is linked directly to the freedom of either avoiding or pursuing reproduction, individuals should have at their disposal the necessary means of fashioning their identities. Thus reproductive technologies are portrayed as neutral instruments assisting individuals in pursuing their reproductive interests. And in order to employ these technologies, procreation must be segmented into the discrete tasks of conception, gestation and child-rearing.

This segmentation initiates the unfolding and enfolding of a reproductive destiny, transforming the focus and context of moral deliberation in its wake. What is lost is an understanding of procreation and child-rearing as an undivided whole, and how specific reproductive decisions should cohere with its inherent integrity. Rather than judging if a particular choice is right or wrong by its fit with the nature and *telos* of procreation, such a determination is made in respect to accomplishing distinct objectives.

This narrowing of deliberative focus recasts what 'right' and 'wrong' come to mean. Within more traditional patterns of deliberation, a choice is assessed in terms of its compatibility or incompatibility with what it means to be a good spouse and parent. Practising the requisite virtues entails that some options cannot be entertained, or, returning to Grant's analogy, pro-creation is part of a package deal whose terms cannot be altered without distorting the normative meaning of marriage and parenthood. In contrast, procreative liberty promotes deliber-ation in which particular choices are assessed in terms of how they assist individuals in pursuing their reproductive interests. Some options are better than others in respect to conception, gestation and child-rearing. A choice is 'right' so long as no person is harmed in achieving a reproductive objective. Thus individuals should not be restricted by the imposed conditions of a package deal in picking and choosing among various options.

It is at this point that procreative liberty fails to recognise that the reproductive choice it propounds is itself a package deal, imposing the constraints of its destiny. In order to exercise certain reproductive options relevant techniques must be deployed, and their design not only delimits the purposes for which they are used, but also shapes what freedom and choosing come to mean. Procreative liberty presupposes a mis-leading understanding of technological neutrality by contending that persons are free to use or not use various techniques to implement their reproductive choices. Robertson could easily paraphrase the reassuring adage of Grant's com-puter scientist that reproductive technology does not impose on us the ways it should be used.

Yet technology does impose its ways upon its users, dis-figuring normative terms and roles in its wake. Purpose becomes an asserted goal rather than a given end, choice becomes a strategy of selecting and discarding options rather than disciplined discernment, and freedom becomes a matter of satisfying personal desires rather than a practice of virtue. When the destiny of procreation is switched from a fruition of marital and parental love to a pursuit of fulfilling one's self-interests, then purpose, choice and freedom take on distinctly different connotations. Although procreative liberty uses qualified accounts of collaborative reproduction, which to greater and lesser extents resemble traditional accounts of marriage and parenthood, they imply differing meanings when torn away from a familial destiny. Instead of seeing procreation as a means of receiving and caring for the gift of a child, it becomes a reproductive project of obtaining a child of one's own. And in doing so, it is difficult to see how such a child cannot be regarded as something other than an artefact or commodity.

Proponents of procreative liberty have little quarrel with the notion that reproductive technology invites us to think about children in new ways, but they claim this invitation should be welcomed as a liberating opportunity rather than resisted as a temptation. Individuals are assisted to become parents, significant roles they would otherwise be forced to forgo. A particular understanding of marriage and parenthood is not necessarily demeaned in assisting persons to satisfy a natural and healthy desire for offspring. In this respect, reproduction is rightfully understood as a worthwhile project facilitating personal fulfilment.

It is with the pejorative imagery of children as commodities that proponents of procreative liberty cry foul. Whether natural or artificial means of pursuing procreation are employed, it is difficult to see a child as other than an outcome of reproductive choices. It is individuals who decide whether or not to become parents, and reproductive technology simply expands the range of options in exercising this choice. Nor does employing the natural method prevent children from being perceived as artefacts. Prior to the advent of reproductive technology, parents produced offspring for the sake of greater economic productivity or security. There is no reason to assume that merely using reproductive technology will commodify children to any greater or lesser extent than did previous generations.

In short, objections that introducing reproductive technologies alter the very nature of procreation and parenthood are
dismissed because they are symbolic rather than substantive,
and are thereby insufficient to restrict individuals from pursuing their reproductive interests. The only substantive
complaint that can be raised is that an act harms a person, and
none of the objections demonstrate that this is the case. Moreover, if some individuals find these objections persuasive they
are at liberty to act accordingly. They are free to treat embryos
or fetuses as persons, to collaborate exclusively with a spouse,
or refrain from employing any artificial techniques. Given a
lack of moral consensus, the beliefs of some individuals cannot
be imposed upon others. Consequently, public moral deliberation must confine itself to procedural issues protecting the
rights of individuals to pursue their reproductive interests,
while ensuring that no persons are harmed in the process.

Symbols, however, play an inescapable role in moral deliberation. Symbols shape both descriptive and interpretative
accounts, thereby determining what is included and excluded
within a range of deliberative considerations. Or as Meilaender
contends, 'symbols do not express thoughts we (privately) have;
they give rise to thought. We cannot think in nonsymbolic
ways.'[37] Proponents of procreative liberty not only fail to admit
the symbolic importance of such terms as 'person', 'freedom'
and 'choice', but also refuse to subject them to any normative
scrutiny in assessing their symbolic adequacy.

Expanding the range of reproductive choice, for instance, is
portrayed as a liberating development for individuals facing
various natural or social constraints. The analogy of a supermarket is preferable to the package deal because the former can
accommodate the latter – old reproductive options are placed
alongside new ones. Yet these traditional choices are now
enfolded within a package deal of picking and choosing. The
very concept of a supermarket not only imposes a particular
perception of how food is produced and distributed, and which
ingredients constitute a normal diet, but also dictates certain
expectations on how consumers should conduct themselves

while shopping. Individuals are not entitled to prevent others from selecting items they may find objectionable, for presumably the shelves are stocked with 'safe' products. A supermarket makes no normative claims about what constitutes a 'good diet', for customers select the items they want. It is important to emphasise that even if a substantial majority opt for ingredients of a 'good diet', they do so *within conditions imposed by the supermarket's package deal of picking and choosing*. Thus the items selected tell us little about the nature of a good diet, but the act of selecting discloses a great deal about what is required to be a good shopper, namely, that there is no objective standard for determining the difference between good and bad choices.

A similar pattern is repeated in Robertson's reproductive supermarket. Not only does an expanding array of 'safe' reproductive options transform a perception of how offspring may be obtained, but a standard of conduct is also imposed upon consumers that individuals are not entitled to prevent others from selecting options they themselves may find objectionable. Procreative liberty makes no normative claims about marriage, parenthood or family, because these roles and institutions may be ignored or redefined in line with an individual's reproductive interests. Juxtaposing old and new options highlights the symbolic importance of choice, for there are no objective criteria differentiating good from bad choices other than avoiding harm. Again it needs to be stressed that even if a substantial majority opts for the traditional preference, they do so *within conditions imposed by a package deal of reproductive choice*. Consequently, what is chosen tells us little about the nature and normative structure of procreation or parenthood, but the act of choosing reveals much about what is required in exercising procreative liberty, namely, that one choice is no better than another except as determined by those individuals pursuing their reproductive interests.

The symbol of reproductive choice is misleading. In reducing parenthood to an expression of will, the resulting choices are not genuinely different options, but differing guises of a common act. Procreative liberty presumes that regardless of what method is employed, pursuing one's reproductive interests always entails some form of commissioning and collaboration. Once an individual determines that it is in her best interest to reproduce, then she commissions a process of obtaining a child in which the extent of collaboration with others is set by the methods (e.g. coitus, adoption, ART) employed to achieve this end. The dominant symbol of choice is accompanied by a destiny of the child as artefact in which the means used to obtain a child are irrelevant, so long as no one collaborating in a reproductive project is harmed.

The symbol of the child as gift, however, initiates the unfolding of a different destiny. God entrusts a child into the care of parents to provide a place of timely belonging. Moreover, there are conditions set for how this gift is to be received in a procreative or charitable manner, so that the destiny of familial fellowship determines the means to be employed. Contrary to proponents of procreative liberty, symbols do matter in moral deliberation, for they shape our perception of what we set out to achieve, and what we may or may not do in achieving it.

One of the most interesting characteristics of a gift is its sheer givenness and gratuitousness. A true gift cannot be begged, borrowed or bought. Pestering someone to buy us something we want or purchasing an item for ourselves is not the same thing as having a gift bestowed upon or entrusted to us. Moreover, a gift carries with it an implied purpose for how it should be used, as well as something of the character and expectations of the giver. If we are given a painting, for instance, we may assume its purpose is to be hung on a wall rather than used to start a fire in the fireplace. In addition, the giver implies some expectation on how an otherwise identical gift is to be used. For example, it is one thing to receive a gun from a skilled hunter, and quite a different matter to receive it from a notorious bank robber.

If we perceive children as gifts entrusted to our care rather than as outcomes of reproductive projects, we confront a different set of concerns in deliberating on the moral uses of reproductive technology. If children are gifts, does this not imply a given and gratuitous structure to the parent–child relationship? And if children are not properly a means of one's self-fulfilment, does this not suggest an unconditional quality to the parent–child relationship that is not premised upon offspring as desirable artefacts? Given the current fixation on the reproductive rights and interests of autonomous persons, these questions cannot be addressed adequately, much less answered, without recourse to much fuller and richer symbols than that of choice.

Returning to the research project that opened this chapter, we may soon be able to use donated eggs to produce offspring genetically related to both parents. Presumably, such an achievement would technically meet the criteria of procreative stewardship, implying that a 'limited' amount of collaboration with a third party is permissible. Such reasoning has already been enfolded into the symbolism and destiny of reproductive choice, however, for it misses the sheer novelty of producing a child who 'technically' has three biological parents. If a vindicated order of creation being drawn toward its destiny in Christ should shape the moral ordering of procreation, then the novelty of this prospect should at least give us some pause if contemplating such 'limited' collaboration has not already transformed our perception of procreation into a reproductive project. Beginning moral deliberation with what is technically feasible is simply to succumb to the package deal of picking and choosing. Rather, if a couple is called by God to become parents, then various technologies must be assessed in terms of how they may assist or prevent these two parents in preparing themselves to receive the gift of children.

The account of procreative stewardship being developed in this book argues in favour of placing extensive restrictions on ART. An important question, however, now demands our attention: to what extent may we use various technologies to prevent the birth of severely ill or disabled children?

....

Robert and Rebecca are in their early forties and have been married a little over a year. Although they married 'late in life', they want to have a child. Both of them, however, carry a recessive gene for cystic fibrosis (CF) which means that their child would run a 25 per cent risk of being affected. They are concerned about being able to provide proper care for a severely ill child, yet the prospect of remaining childless is equally distressing. They are also concerned that their age could work against them if they attempt to adopt, and employing IVF using donated eggs or sperm makes them uncomfortable, since the resulting child would not be genetically related to both of them.

Rebecca and Robert learn about a procedure called preimplantation genetic diagnosis (PGD), which if used in conjunction with IVF could prevent the birth of a child affected by CF. Although such a technique would alleviate many of their health-care worries, they are concerned about its morality and wonder if they should just accept their 'sad fate'. They turn to their pastor for advice. If you were their pastor, what counsel would you offer?

chapter five

Quality Control and Experimentation

This chapter examines the extent to which humans may intervene in the reproductive process in order to prevent the birth of a child with a severely deleterious disease or disability. The first section provides an overview of current quality-control techniques and research policies concerning the use of embryos. The second section summarises various positions on quality-control techniques and experiments utilising embryos. The following sections argue that faithfully exercising procreative stewardship permits a highly restricted employment of quality-control techniques and use of embryos within research protocols.

RECENT TECHNOLOGICAL ADVANCES not only assist the human reproductive process, but also enable us to exert greater control over its outcomes. Within an expanding range of diagnostic parameters, we can prevent the birth of children with severely debilitating illnesses or disabilities. Moreover, experiments performed on embryos may spur the development of more effective therapies along a wide spectrum of diseases. Consequently, the advent of *quality-control* techniques is hailed as a blessing, preventing children (as well as their parents) from enduring unnecessary suffering. More importantly, perhaps, by combining these techniques with our growing knowledge of the genetic components of many illnesses and disabilities, we may be taking our first step into a new era of more effective health care.

The ability to exert quality control over human reproduction raises a number of troubling concerns. There are issues concerning the parent–child relationship. To what extent, for instance, should parents select the genetic traits of offspring? There are issues involving the exploitation of human life at its earliest stages of development. Is it permissible, for example, to conduct experiments on unneeded or discarded embryos, or harvest stem cells from aborted fetuses?

These troubling concerns, however, are accompanied by a number of important considerations. Parents are obliged to promote the health of their children. To what extent may parental care be exhibited at antenatal stages of development? Healthy individuals also promote the common good. To what extent may quality-control techniques be employed to prevent chronic conditions requiring prolonged and expensive medical care? And to what extent may embryos and fetuses be used to develop more effective therapies?

In examining these questions we will first explore the natural and understandable desire of parents for healthy offspring, revisit the quality-control techniques currently available, and summarise public policies governing research on antenatal forms of life. This is followed by a survey of representative positions on the ethics of quality-control and antenatal research. The chapter concludes with an assessment of quality-control techniques and antenatal research within a framework of procreative stewardship. It should also be noted that attention is restricted to issues preventing deleterious or undesirable traits in offspring, excluding the important but more speculative questions concerning the enhancement of desirable traits, which will become practically significant if and when such technological capabilities become feasible.

Parental hopes and fears

A parental desire for healthy children is certainly natural and understandable. Most parents want what is best for offspring, and will sacrifice their own interests to give their children the best possible start in life. Parents are rightfully anxious when their son or daughter becomes seriously ill. Indeed, good parents do all that is in their power to prevent their children from suffering needlessly. Prospective parents 'hoping' for a severely ill or disabled child, for instance, or parents withholding standard medical care from their children, are generally regarded as incompetent or negligent.

To what extent may parents exhibit such care at the antenatal stage? If it were possible to prevent a child from being born with such debilitating diseases as cystic fibrosis or Down's syndrome, would not a loving parent be expected, or even obliged to do so? Or posed more prosaically: what loving or responsible parent would withhold good health from their children?

For previous generations these questions were merely hypothetical. There was little parents could do concerning the health of offspring until after birth, and even then there were distinct limits on what medicine could accomplish. To date, for example, there are no cures for cystic fibrosis or Down's syndrome. Too often parents, as well as physicians, could provide little more than comfort and company for children born with debilitating illnesses or disabilities. Individuals who were known to be at risk of passing on inherited diseases were often urged either not to marry, or to forgo procreation, or to adopt rather than play the game of genetic roulette.

With the advent of quality-control techniques, however, parents could, in some instances, spare children from needless suffering. As was examined in the first chapter, there are fetal monitoring devices, such as amniocentesis and CVS, that can disclose a number of deleterious conditions. In addition, embryo testing and screening prior to implantation (PGD) is now available for an expanding range of diseases. Moreover, with improved diagnostic accuracy and the knowledge being gained from the Human Genome Project (HGP), parents will have greater assurance that they will not be subjecting offspring to unnecessary risks.

We must be clear, however, that at present quality-control techniques do not prevent a deleterious condition from occurring in a particular child. Rather, these techniques *prevent the birth of a child manifesting an unwanted or undesirable trait*. In the absence of effective antenatal or postnatal therapies, affected fetuses are often aborted, or affected embryos discarded. The most efficacious method of sparing a child unnecessary suffering is to terminate a pregnancy or refuse to implant an embryo.

It is not surprising that quality-control techniques have generated hotly contested disputes, given highly disparate assessments over the moral status of antenatal forms of life and what legal safeguards should be in place protecting them. Even the most ardent champions of procreative liberty admit that although embryos and fetuses are not persons, they should nonetheless not be treated in a cavalier manner but should be shown respect. Consequently, many countries have enacted policies or guidelines governing the use of quality-control techniques.

In the United Kingdom, for example, an abortion may be performed if there is a 'substantial' risk of fetal abnormality that will be likely to result in a 'serious handicap', or jeopardise a child's 'long term survival' following birth.[1] The criteria used for determining the likelihood of a serious handicap include: availability of effective *in utero* or postnatal treatments, self-awareness and communication abilities, extent of suffering, and lack of independence.[2] In addition, an abortion may be performed to safeguard a pregnant woman's physical, mental or social well-being.

The Human Fertilisation and Embryology Authority (HFEA) was established in 1991 to regulate reproductive technologies and oversee human embryo research. PGD falls under the purview of HFEA guidelines. As was discussed in the first chapter, PGD may be used to test embryos for various genetic and chromosomal disorders. The range of 'serious disorders' that can be diagnosed include Down's syndrome, cystic fibrosis, Duchenne muscular dystrophy, haemophilia, Huntington's disease, sickle cell disease, and a number of uncommon cancers. Potentially, PGD could also be applied to identify risk for late onset conditions such as some forms of heart disease, diabetes and more common cancers.[3]

The HFEA has acknowledged a 'public unease' accompanying recent medical and scientific advances, recognising that 'PGD forms part of a complex debate on genetics and the use of genetic information'. Consequently, in conjunction with the Advisory Committee on Genetic Testing (ACGT), a working group was commissioned to review current guidelines and practices for the purpose of establishing 'an appropriate ethical framework'.[4]

There are a number of clinical and practical problems associated with PGD. Misdiagnosis may occur through either technical failure or sampling unrepresentative cells. Several biopsies need to be performed to reduce misdiagnosis, resulting in fewer embryos available for implantation when combined with affected or damaged embryos. Given the low success rate of IVF, a woman may have to undergo multiple IVF cycles to improve the chances of pregnancy. Moreover, the 'longer term effects of embryo biopsy on child development are unknown', and since PGD is an expensive procedure access may be restricted 'by the ability of patients to meet the costs themselves, or by the willingness of health authorities to fund the treatment'.[5]

The working group admits that PGD may inspire a prejudicial climate against children (as well as their parents) with what are perceived to be 'preventable' genetic disabilities. Yet the working group insists that if parents are 'given the choice [that] it would be better for a child to be free of a serious disease', exercising this option 'does not necessarily reflect on attitudes towards people with that disease'. In order to prevent such stigmatisation, the working group recommends that PGD be restricted to preventing a 'serious medical condition' rather than identifying 'social or psychological characteristics'. In addition, many individuals may find PGD preferable to other diagnostic options (e.g. amniocentesis or CVS) because it involves the destruction of embryos rather than fetuses. The working group acknowledges that defining what constitutes a 'serious disorder' is a highly challenging prospect, given the variability of severity among affected children and ability of parents to cope or provide care. Yet the working group insists that PGD offers a viable option 'to families who have to make difficult choices where there is a risk that their children may be affected'. Moreover, each 'family should be free to make their own choices . . . and their view will be one of the most important determining factors in assessing the justification for PGD'.[6]

The working group's document raises the issue of replacing carrier or affected embryos. On the one hand, an embryo may not be affected by a particular genetic disorder, but nonetheless carry the trait that can be subsequently passed on to offspring. For example, if a person carrying the recessive gene for cystic fibrosis mates with another carrier, there is a one-in-four chance that offspring will be affected. On the other hand, in some instances a couple may request PGD treatment in order to produce an affected embryo. For example, a congenitally deaf couple may believe that 'a child with normal hearing would be alienated from their environment and that this would be harmful to both the child and the couple'. These scenarios raise a larger issue of the extent to which physicians and clinicians should assist the birth of a child with a genetic disorder, especially given the legal requirement that the welfare of the child must be taken into account before treatment is approved.[7]

In addition, the working group addresses the question of using PGD to test for late onset disorders and predisposition for certain conditions. An individual may be affected by a genetic disorder that is not expressed for many years or even decades. In some cases, such as Huntington's disease, debilitating illness and premature death is certain. In other cases, such as certain forms of breast cancer, a risk factor can be identified but it is unknown if a particular individual will develop the disease. Furthermore, the severity of many conditions cannot be predicted in advance, and 'late' onset may range from early childhood to middle age depending on the condition in question. With anticipated advances in genetic research, testing an embryo for a predisposition toward a certain disease may soon be available. Such testing would indicate that a particular genetic predisposition in conjunction with certain environmental factors and lifestyle could lead to the onset of such debilitating conditions as Alzheimer's disease and some forms of coronary heart disease. Should the presence of late-onset or predisposition factors disqualify an embryo from being implanted? The working group's document offers no objective standards for making this determination. Rather, it suggests that such an assessment will vary among individuals, families and the condition in question, incorporating a wide range of considerations and quality of life judgements.[8]

The HFEA also regulates research conducted on human embryos 'outside the body'. Such research is vital to ensure continuing medical advances. To secure a research licence it must be demonstrated that the use of human embryos is 'necessary or desirable' for one of the following reasons:

- promoting the treatment of infertility;
- gaining additional knowledge about the causes of miscarriages or congenital disease;
- developing more effective contraception;
- developing more effective methods for detecting genetic or chromosomal abnormalities in embryos prior to implantation.

Embryos used for research must be 'obtained with appropriate consent', and cannot be used for any purposes other than those specified in the licence. It is forbidden to use or keep an embryo past the fourteenth day of development or appearance of the 'primitive streak', or to place it in an animal. In addition, the nucleus of a cell from a human embryo may not be removed and replaced with the nucleus from another person or embryo, nor may the genetic structure of a cell be altered within an embryo.[9]

The stated purpose of public policy guidelines, such as those propounded by the HFEA, is to provide an ethical framework governing research and the use of quality-control techniques in a manner that 'respects' human embryos. Yet how moral questions are identified, posed and addressed often hides underlying philosophical and ideological presuppositions that shape the course of subsequent moral deliberation. It is toward investigating this philosophical and ideological substructure that we now turn our attention.

Desirable and undesirable children

As was discussed previously, the central tenet of procreative liberty is that every person has a right to pursue his or her reproductive interests. If a person has a right to obtain a child, then he or she also has an interest in obtaining a desirable child. Consequently, few restrictions should be placed on quality-control techniques, the only provisos being that embryos should be treated with respect, and offspring should not be made 'less healthy or whole than they could be'.[10] Moreover, employing quality-control techniques may be seen as an expression of parental care in which parents are taking responsible steps to prevent their children from unnecessary suffering; they are doing what any good parent would do, namely, providing their children with the best possible start in life. The destruction of embryos necessitated by quality-control techniques and experimentation is permissible since no person is purportedly harmed, and the results are in turn beneficial to children and their parents.

The HFEA guidelines presumably ensure a respect for embryos by requiring that quality-control techniques be restricted to preventing only 'serious' disorders, and specifying which experimental procedures can and cannot be performed.

Expanding the range of quality-control options, however, provides the bedrock of these guidelines, and experimentation with embryos is justified largely by its potential to offer reproductive options. The primacy of the interests and rights of autonomous persons is ensconced in the manner in which the ethical issues are presented and discussed.

One consequence of this presumption is that it skews the course of public moral deliberation by focusing almost exclusively on procedural questions of access and research guidelines. The principal issue at stake, using the distinction that was made by H. Tristram Engelhardt in Chapter 1, is what persons 'in a strict sense' can and cannot do to or with persons 'in a social sense' (embryos) to avoid the birth of undesirable children. Normative claims, other than the primacy of autonomous persons, are not admitted into the process of formulating an 'appropriate ethical framework'. If the beliefs of some individuals prevent them from using quality-control techniques, their preference can be accommodated within procedures protecting their choices. In short, such public policy deliberations are often exercises in setting minimal rules for controlling the qualitative outcomes of various reproductive projects. Such an exercise not only shapes the terms of public moral debate but may also influence how Christian normative claims are formulated and argued.

One approach might be to insist that it is wrong to withhold the rights and protections enjoyed by autonomous persons from embryos. Embryos should be afforded such rights and protections in virtue of their status as members of the human species. Consequently, as *Donum Vitae* and Germain Grisez contend, every embryo has a fundamental right to life and should not be destroyed for the sake of avoiding an undesirable child or conducting research.[11]

In a similar vein, Paul Ramsey argues that quality-control techniques and most research protocols involving embryos violate the central tenets of medicine, namely, consent and beneficence. Embryos cannot consent to the procedures they are subjected to, nor do embryos derive any direct benefit from their participation in experiments conducted upon them. Although it may be objected that parents make medical decisions on behalf of their dependent children, this role does not entitle them to sacrifice less desirable siblings in order to retain a more desirable child. In addition, parents may not subject their children to experimental treatments from which they will enjoy no benefit and which will surely end in their death.[12]

D. Gareth Jones plots a middle course between the embryo as person or tissue, arguing that it should be treated as a potential person. Although embryos should be accorded high levels of respect and protection, this does not entitle them to an inherent right to life. The high rate of natural 'pregnancy wastage', often caused by genetic abnormalities, suggests that assigning any personal status to embryos would prove a mysterious and problematic proposition from which no obvious moral principles or guidelines can be drawn. In addition, embryos should not be perceived as any more or less 'innocent' than other forms of human life, thereby making them suitable subjects for scientific research provided there are adequate safeguards.[13]

James Gustafson purportedly rejects any sharp distinction between accounts of personhood in a strict or social sense, because the principal metaphors used to describe a person invariably appeal to both natural and social categories. Nonetheless, a person is an agent possessing a capacity to undertake a certain course of action in line with particular intentions or purposes. Consequently, persons (agents) should be guided by the principle that human life should be preserved rather than destroyed, especially in regard to those who cannot assert a right to life (e.g. embryos), although there are always exceptions to this rule.[14]

More radically, Joseph Fletcher asserts that 'neocortical function' is the 'essential trait' of personhood, and no binding moral obligations are owed to humans lacking this criterion. Thus a virtually unrestricted range of quality-control techniques and experimental procedures may be performed.[15]

Stanley Hauerwas takes a different approach by focusing on the role medicine should play rather than attempting to resolve the thorny issues involving personhood. The primary purpose of medicine is not necessarily to prevent suffering. This is especially the case when the only means of preventing suffering is to destroy the 'patient', as in the case of an affected embryo. Rather, the purpose of medicine is to provide a link between the 'sick' and 'healthy', ensuring that the latter will not abandon the former. In treating an illness or disability, medicine is an important link in maintaining a fellowship between a community and those who suffer. This commitment to keeping company with the suffering is particularly pronounced in a parent–child relationship.[16]

According to Hauerwas, procedural disputes over the ethics of quality control and experimentation prove unsatisfactory because they are based on liberal principles that are doomed to fail. Procreative liberty, for instance, simply presumes that medicine is a useful tool enabling autonomous persons to pursue their reproductive interests. Thus the only significant moral challenge is to establish procedures maximising a free pursuit of these interests, and ensuring that other persons will not be harmed in the process. Since it is in the interest of parents to obtain desirable, or at least avoid undesirable, offspring, access to quality-control techniques should not be restricted unduly.

Yet as Hauerwas contends, medicine incorporates an illiberal presupposition inhibiting autonomy, namely, that patients submit themselves to the care of physicians who constrain their freedom in pursuing good health. Patients and physicians share a vision of what good health means, but play different roles in pursuing this common end. The structure of this relationship delineates a moral practice of medicine. As Hauerwas argues, autonomy is a last resort in late liberal society that can draw no integral relation among various goods. A moral practice of medicine, however, requires some agreement on what goods a community should pursue. The authority of medicine depends on a community with an established ordering of goods, and in its absence such authority cannot be 'vindicated or sustained'.

Since autonomy cannot provide an adequate basis for such authority, is a more reliable foundation available? For Hauerwas, the human body provides such an alternative.[17] In learning to live within a structure of bodily limitations, the desires of patients and application of medical treatments are set accordingly. Medicine is the practice of enabling humans to live an embodied existence, submitting their respective skills and desires as physicians and patients to the authority of the body's natural structure. This emphasis on the embodied character of human life may appear obvious, but it is often overlooked or discounted in contemporary moral deliberation. In amplifying the primacy of the autonomous will, medicine perceives the body not as the source of its authority but an obstacle to be overcome, promoting a dualism in which embodied personhood is subsumed into an assertive, dis-embodied will. This dualism becomes more pronounced when embryos are used as resources in obtaining a desirable child.

What is lost in this dualism is the acknowledgement that human life is commenced and lived out as embodied creatures in fellowship with other embodied creatures. The structures of these associations, like the structure of the body, have inherent natures that are disregarded at the cost of diminishing the basic sources of human flourishing. Respecting the character of embodied life does not imply that humans may be reduced to the sum total of biological processes. Rather, such respect affirms the role biology plays in ordering human lives.

The authority of the body is a reminder that medicine is itself a moral practice serving the end of ordering human lives within their various associations, and it is this embodied character that should shape the practice of medicine. Medicine rightfully intervenes in biological processes, assisting humans in dis-charging their duties and responsibilities. Yet such intervention takes its principal cues from the body instead of the will. Respecting the authority of the body entails a normative prac-tice of medicine, honouring the social structures of human life.

Medicine, for instance, should take into account the nature of marriage and family to assist individuals in exercising their parental responsibilities, rather than aiding autonomous persons to overcome imposed biological and social constraints.

Although there are some distinct problems with Hauerwas' accounts of suffering and the authority of the body, he nonetheless provides helpful themes that can be built upon in assessing what role, if any, quality control plays within a framework of procreative stewardship.

Healthy babies and perfect babies

Does procreative stewardship encompass parental responsibilities regarding the health of offspring? May these responsibilities be exercised through antenatal interventions?[18] These questions may be answered affirmatively, provided such interventions are guided by reasonable expectations and inherent limitations. It is reasonable for parents to promote antenatal development by refraining from activities endangering a fetus. Medicine assists parents by disclosing conditions that, in some instances, can be treated either before or following birth.

There are, however, limits to the extent that antenatal interventions can or should be undertaken. It is unrealistic to assume that parents can protect children from every harm. Moreover, such an expectation fails to acknowledge that the character of familial belonging is not to prevent potential threats to one's personal well-being, but to provide strength and support in facing adversity. Medicine disables procreative stewardship when quality control is used to obtain a 'perfect baby' rather than to promote the health of a particular child.

Since promoting the health of offspring at the antenatal stage is a proper dimension of procreative stewardship, and since medicine may assist parents in discharging this responsibility, then a *limited employment of quality-control techniques is permissible, provided their use accords with the nature, structure and* telos *of the spheres in which procreation is pursued or assisted.* Three general parameters set these limitations.

First, employing a quality-control technique should not diminish a sense of *unconditional belonging* between parents and children. The intention is not to satisfy a parental longing for a desirable child, but to prevent a severe illness or disability, substantially incapacitating the parent–child relationship. This parameter acknowledges the difference in the parent–child relationship at the antenatal and postnatal stages, while preventing it from becoming an overriding factor. When a child is very ill, for example, parents suffer distress, but the object of their concern is the health of, rather than their relationship with, their child. With an unborn child who is ill, however, the situation is different because it pre-dates a critical familial bonding. Although this lack of familial bonding may permit more invasive treatment, it does not imply that parents may employ any available means to prevent a potentially distressing or undesirable situation regarding their care of offspring following birth.

Second, employing a quality-control technique should not violate the *embodied character* of procreation. A legitimate attempt to spare a child from illness or disability is not synonymous with bypassing a couple's genes or enhancing the chances of passing on the most desirable traits. The purpose of exerting limited quality control is to prevent the birth of a severely ill child and not to pre-select the most desirable one.

Third, employing a quality-control technique should be guided by a practice of medicine submitting itself to the *authority of the body*. Such a practice takes its principal cues from the bodies of parents and developing offspring rather than the desires of individuals manipulating the qualitative outcomes of reproductive projects. Submitting procreation to the authority of the body recognises that its pursuit is more akin to a couple preparing themselves to receive the gift of a child than making a baby as a desirable artefact. Moreover, the application of these three parameters should accord with the covenants of mutual trust and fidelity between child and parents, wife and husband, patient and physician, reflecting the normative structure and *telos* of these respective relationships.

Given these parameters there are a number of quality-control techniques that are permissible because they respect the nature of familial belonging, the embodied character of procreation and the authority of the body. A couple carrying a deleterious genetic trait may refrain from sexual intercourse, or employ contraceptive or sterilisation techniques. During pregnancy a regimen of diet and rest, as well as avoiding hazardous environments, can be followed. A fetus may be monitored, tested and treated if appropriate therapies are available. Genetic testing and screening of embryos may also be used, provided their purpose is clearly therapeutic rather than to select or enhance desirable traits.

It is admittedly difficult to draw a sharp distinction between genetic therapy and enhancement. In some respects, therapy is an enhancement since the restoration of health is an improvement over ill health. Yet there is a difference between employing a technique to treat a severe illness or disability, and selecting or enhancing characteristics that would give offspring certain social advantages. Replacing a defective gene causing cystic fibrosis, for example, is not the same as enhancing physical stature or intelligence in a society where people of short stature or low intelligence suffer unjust discrimination. Although the distinction between therapy and selection or enhancement is ambiguous, it nonetheless provides a useful conceptual tool for drawing the boundaries of obligation and tolerance.[19]

The limits implied by this distinction may be made more explicit by examining three borderline cases:

- the testing and selective implantation of embryos;
- cloning embryos for implantation;
- monitoring and selectively aborting fetuses.

For the sake of argument, it is assumed that in each case a couple is known to be carrying a genetic trait that is likely to cause a severely debilitating illness or disability, and there are no effective therapies for treating the condition. Although it is notoriously difficult to set an objective standard for measuring severity, it is again assumed, for the sake of argument, that such criteria could be established. For the sake of simplicity, it is assumed that the onset of the condition in question will occur at or shortly after birth.

Most importantly, no position on when personhood begins is assumed or argued. These borderline cases are used as a means of enquiring into the extent that quality-control techniques may be employed by parents, exercising their procreative stewardship, in the absence of any consensus regarding the inherent or assigned status of antenatal life. This is not to suggest that the issue of whether or not an embryo is a person is unimportant. Rather, the purpose of this exercise is to demonstrate that even in the absence of a consensus regarding the personhood of an embryo normative claims can nonetheless be made and argued. The intent is to sketch out the contours of a mode of deliberation based on a normative structure and *telos* of the family, procreation and medicine in contrast to those based on the reproductive interests and rights of autonomous persons.

Testing and selective implantation of embryos

This treatment entails IVF using spouses' gametes in which a number of embryos are produced and tested for the deleterious gene in question. Unaffected embryos are implanted in the wife's womb while affected ones are discarded. A case for employing this treatment may be made along the following lines: there are rare genetically related illnesses or disabilities which if inherited by offspring may virtually preclude any significant development of the parent–child relationship following birth. Since parents are responsible for promoting the health of their children, they may use these techniques to prevent passing on a severely debilitating condition, provided there are no effective therapies available. This technique is a provisional measure until such time as effective therapies are developed. Consequently, severity should be defined in a manner promoting a shrinking, instead of expanding, list of conditions for which testing and selectively implanting embryos are warranted.

It may be objected that testing and selectively implanting embryos fall beyond the parameters outlined above. These techniques pervert the unconditional nature of familial belonging into a conditional genetic criterion. Children are admitted to a family only if they pass a test, destroying the fabric of an unfolding and expansive familial love. A genetic trait jeopardising the quality of the parent–child relationship should not disqualify an embryo from subsequent development or parental care. Furthermore, these techniques disregard the authority of the body. Carrying a deleterious trait is a bodily limitation imposed on a couple pursuing procreation. By destroying affected embryos medicine dismisses their potential for embodied life, albeit diminished, thereby submitting itself to the wilful desire of parents to sever their relationship with undesirable offspring. More troubling still is that these techniques violate the embodied character of procreation. Even if IVF may be used to assist procreation, this does not permit selecting which embryos shall or shall not be implanted. Introducing qualitative criteria transforms procreation into a reproductive project. Although there is a degree of natural wastage of embryos, it is an inherent element of procreation that is not rightfully subject to wilful manipulation.

In reply, it is conceded that using qualitative criteria introduces a potentially troubling consideration. The embodied character of procreation is perverted in this instance only if these techniques are used to select the most desirable embryo among a range of possible candidates. The question of intent is paramount in this discussion, because the purpose is not to obtain the most desirable child possible but to prevent offspring from inheriting a deleterious trait within a narrow range of diagnostic indications. If this end is to be achieved in the absence of effective therapies, then the destruction of affected embryos is a necessary, though regrettable and foreseen, consequence. The objection is correct in noting that a degree of wilfulness is introduced, but it cannot be known in advance whether selecting embryos for implantation within a narrow range of diagnostic criteria will prove any less 'moral' than natural selection. Although testing and selectively implanting embryos diminishes the embodied structure of procreation, its nature and *telos* are not sufficiently violated to prohibit qualitative interventions into a restricted range of debilitating conditions.

Given this limited purpose, neither do these techniques ignore the authority of the body. Instead of bypassing potentially defective genes by using donated gametes, medical attention is focused on expediting what may be considered the death of a dying embryo. The intent is not to prevent the birth of undesirable offspring, but an attempt to prevent the birth of a mortally and incurably ill child. This situation is, from the parents' perspective 'undesirable', but avoiding it is not the goal or decisive feature which authorises their intervention. Rather, it is the extreme ill health of offspring that prompts their action. Given narrow diagnostic indications, it is difficult to see how the authority of the body is ignored, unless one is prepared to argue that a child inheriting a deleterious trait is a good result of the couple's procreative stewardship. It is equally difficult to imagine that parents would want, or not object to, their children suffering the consequences of inheriting a deleterious trait because it is a characteristic of the couple's embodied lives.

Testing and selectively implanting embryos perverts the nature of unconditional familial belonging only if used for one of the following purposes: first, if it is employed to create a relatively large number of embryos to be tested for a range of traits from which parents may select the 'best ones' for implantation. Familial belonging then becomes conditional upon offspring meeting a parental checklist. Second, if these techniques are used in lieu of therapeutic treatments because they are less costly or arduous. Familial belonging then becomes conditional upon a child not imposing an unwanted burden.

The objection fails to acknowledge that within a restricted diagnostic context the purpose of embryo selection is not to exclude offspring, but to prevent the further development of an already mortally ill embryo whose birth would virtually preclude any parent–child relationship. It is also because of the absence of this impending mortality that 'carrier' embryos should not be replaced by unaffected ones. The objection is correct in insisting that the quality of the parent–child relationship is not the overriding consideration, but neither is it an irrelevant concern. Even if it is agreed that a substantial number of deleterious traits should not disqualify embryos from being implanted, there is nonetheless a range of conditions that preclude the development of a parent–child relationship. If it is likely that treating such a condition would require relatively brief or prolonged care that is predominantly palliative rather than parental in character, then it is difficult to assert that the antenatal development and birth of such a child enables a couple to establish a familial covenant.

Cloning embryos for implantation

An embryo containing between four and sixteen cells can be divided or split with both halves having the potential for further antenatal development. Such a procedure could be used as a quality-control technique. Imagine the following scenario: in the first IVF cycle only one unaffected embryo is produced. Two or three embryos are usually implanted, given the low success rate. Rather than freezing the embryo and subjecting the woman to an additional cycle, may the embryo be split or cloned to secure additional ones? A negative answer may be formulated along the following lines. Cloning an embryo violates the embodied character of procreation. Whether fertilisation occurs within a woman's body or a test tube, conception entails the creation of a unique genome. Employing this technique also discounts the authority of the body since the gametes of spouses are bypassed in replicating an existing genome.

It may be countered that given the preceding discussion on the testing and selective implantation of embryos this objection is unfounded. There is little significant difference between the two techniques when the intention of implanting the clones of an unaffected embryo is to prevent offspring from inheriting a deleterious genetic trait. What is seemingly being decried is the wilful creation of identical twins or triplets. Yet creating identical twins or triplets no more violates the embodied character of procreation, or the authority of the body, than does the creation of unaffected embryos using two or more IVF cycles. Nor is the wilfulness involved any more telling than in selectively implanting embryos, because the intention is not to obtain identical twins or triplets but to prevent offspring from inheriting a deleterious trait. Moreover, cloning an embryo does not imperil the unconditional nature of familial belonging. In the unlikely event that identical twins or triplets are born it is no more disquieting than if this same outcome occurs through natural procreation, or in the birth of fraternal twins or triplets if selective implantation is used.

In reply to this objection, I agree that the birth of identical (or fraternal) twins or triplets does not violate the inherent nature, structure or *telos* of procreation, medicine or the familial belonging. The degree of wilfulness entailed in splitting or cloning an embryo, however, is more significant than the preceding objection admits. Following the embodied character of procreation, an embryo created in a woman's body, or a test tube, cannot be willed into dividing into twins or triplets. With cloning the clinician is doing more than assisting conception.

Moreover, the intent of cloning is not, strictly speaking, to create an unaffected embryo but to replicate an existing one. Procreation takes on the quality of manufacturing unaffected embryos rather than assisting a couple in begetting healthy offspring, compromising the inherent nature of familial belonging. For if it is permissible to clone an existing embryo to prevent ill health in offspring, then it is also permissible to clone an existing child for the same reason, if and when nuclear-transfer technology ever becomes a safe and reliable technique. A couple discovers, for example, that they carry a severely deleterious genetic trait after the birth of their first child who is unaffected. They want an additional child, but rather than enduring a burdensome process of testing and selectively implanting unaffected embryos they clone their existing child. Despite the couple's humane intention, such a mode of reproduction reduces a child or embryo to a template for siblings, imposing a conditional qualification for familial belonging, namely, that a child posses a particular collection of genes. In short, promoting the health of children does not justify displacing an embodied, though medically assisted, pursuit of procreation with replicating an existing genome.

Monitoring and selective abortion of fetuses

This quality-control technique involves monitoring and aborting a fetus affected by a debilitating illness or disability. The issue in question is not the morality of abortion per se, but interjecting additional qualitative criteria beyond a restricted set of circumstances permitting or indicating an abortion.[20] An argument against employing this technique may be made along the following lines. Aborting an affected fetus violates the nature of unconditional familial belonging. Unlike selective implantation, in which mortally ill embryos are not implanted and are allowed to die, abortion involves the wilful destruction of a fetus. The former marks a parental response to a terminal condition, while the latter represents a withdrawal of parental care. Aborting a fetus under these circumstances also violates the embodied character of procreation because it disrupts a continuity of parental care, separating reproduction from child-rearing as two different spheres, governed by differing sets of interests and responsibilities. In addition, the authority of the body is negated, for rather than attempting to treat a fetus or ameliorate its condition following birth, the fetus is destroyed, eliminating a need for treatment.

It may be objected that prohibiting selective abortion is inconsistent with the previous position on selective implantation, because the intent and consequence are identical. In both instances the intent is to prevent the birth of a severely ill child, and both involve the destruction of affected forms of antenatal life, albeit at different stages of development. Unless an ontological claim regarding the status of a fetus, as opposed to an embryo, is being invoked, there is little difference in destroying either one if they are affected by the same deleterious trait. Such a claim is implied in drawing a morally significant distinction between parental obligations owed to a non-implanted embryo as opposed to a fetus. Yet if a disguised, as well as dubious, argument is being introduced that personhood begins with implantation, then we must also reappraise selective implantation and embryo cloning in respect to this claim.

The objection is correct in noting that arguing for the origin of personhood at the point of implantation would be a dubious undertaking. No such claim is being made in this case against abortion as a quality-control technique. The argument is based entirely on the nature of familial belonging and continuity of parental care entailed in the embodied character of procreation and child-rearing. A significant threshold is reached at implantation, for with gestation there is a relationship between child and parents that did not exist previously. During pregnancy there is a mutual disclosing of this relationship, and a covenant of familial fidelity is initiated. Moreover, the bond of this covenant is formed 'in relationship' rather than based on a 'capacity for relationship'.[21] Given the terms of this covenant, parents are not entitled to use abortion as a way of exercising an option they would have selected prior to implantation, if only they had known then what they know now. Even if following birth the parent–child relationship is devoid of any reciprocity, and even if parents can do nothing more than authorise medical or palliative care, it nonetheless marks a chapter, albeit tragic, in charting a familial history within the uncertain nature of procreation. Consequently, irrespective of when personhood begins, there is a moral difference between indirectly selecting embryos and directly selecting fetuses for destruction.

These borderline cases suggest that, even in the absence of agreement as to when personhood begins, normative concepts derived from procreative stewardship can nonetheless be invoked in deliberating on the morality of quality-control techniques. Yet may such guidelines as the embodied character of procreation, familial belonging and the authority of the body guide our thinking about the morality of conducting research on embryos?

Procreative stewardship and experimentation

Seemingly some position on when personhood begins must be invoked in order to deliberate on the morality of conducting research on embryos. If one believes that personhood begins at conception, for instance, then virtually any experimentation is precluded since it results in the destruction of a person. If, however, one believes that personhood is not present or cannot be assigned until a certain point of antenatal development is reached (e.g. the fourteenth day of development as specified in HFEA guidelines), then a limited range of experimental procedures is permissible so long as certain safeguards are honoured.

Without recourse to a position on when personhood begins, procreative stewardship seemingly hits an inevitable and irresolvable dilemma in respect to experimentation. On the one hand, parents are responsible for promoting the health of offspring. Thus embryo testing and selective implantation within narrowly defined diagnostic parameters is permissible as a provisional measure until such time as effective therapies for treating a severely debilitating condition in question are available. Yet the only way effective therapies can be developed is to conduct research on affected embryos in order to know more about the causes and potential treatments. On the other hand, attempting to apply the structure of the parent–child relationship in an analogous manner to embryos would virtually preclude conducting the research needed to develop effective therapies. It would be immoral for a parent to allow a child to be subjected to medical experiments surely resulting in her death. Procreative stewardship seemingly leads to the contradiction of being simultaneously committed to producing effective therapies and forbidding the necessary means for developing them.

If we revisit the principal themes examined in the previous section, however, we will discover that the dilemma is not irresolvable. First, the embodied character of procreation does not imply that it always results in a good end that we should seek to achieve. At times the natural reproductive process goes awry, resulting in a severe illness or disability that we ought not commend. We cannot say that a good end of procreation is the birth of a mortally ill child.

Second, the authority of the body does not preclude intervening in human biology in order to restore or attain good health. The risk of inheriting a deleterious genetic trait from one's parents is part of our life as embodied creatures, yet this is not a fate to which we must be resigned. Rather, we may take measures to restore proper biological or bodily functions. It is because of the authority of the body that effectively treating a severely debilitating condition is ultimately preferable to bypassing the causes, either through gamete donation or the provisional measure of testing and selectively implanting embryos.

Third, the nature of familial belonging requires that parents promote the health of offspring. As was argued in the previous section, this parental responsibility may be exercised during antenatal stages of development. Moreover, it was argued that more intrusive interventions are permissible prior to implantation, if the intent is to prevent further development of an embryo that will be likely to result in the birth of a mortally ill child. Thus subjecting an affected embryo to experiments surely resulting in its destruction is not analogous to the relationship between a mortally ill child and her parents.

Consequently, experimentation conducted on affected embryos is permissible, provided the research is conducted for the purpose of gaining knowledge with potentially diagnostic or therapeutic applications regarding the condition being examined. As was the case with highly restricted uses of quality-control techniques, the purpose of such experimentation is not to destroy embryos or produce more desirable children. Rather, the intent is to develop effective therapies in which the destruction of affected embryos is a regrettable and foreseeable consequence. In short, the goal is to develop therapies that will render the provisional quality-control technique of testing and selectively implanting embryos unnecessary.

In making this case for experimentation within narrowly defined diagnostic parameters, two important clarifications must be stressed: first, it is not arguing that, since affected embryos will be destroyed, there is no reason for not gaining some benefit by using them as research subjects. The medical knowledge gained from such experiments would at least mitigate a tragic set of circumstances; an affected embryo would not be destroyed in vain. An attempt to mitigate a tragedy, however, does not justify acts that under 'normal' circumstances would be judged immoral or improper. We do not condone, by way of analogy, personal vengeance because it might help victims mitigate the tragedy of a crime committed against them. Moreover, such a justification for experimentation might set a precedent in which similar arguments could be applied in 'tragic' circumstances involving unwanted embryos, aborted fetuses or terminally ill infants.

Second, some theologians contend that since all humans are fallen creatures, embryos (as well as fetuses and children) should not be perceived as being inherently 'innocent'. Such a view romanticises antenatal life, arbitrarily cut off from the larger human community. Since all humans are 'conceived' within a fallen world, they may also participate in various human endeavours, such as scientific research, without the encumbrance of overly stringent protections virtually precluding their participation. What this argument fails to recognise, however, is that our common 'fallen condition' does not relieve us from the burden of making judgements regarding relative states of 'innocence' or 'guilt'. Even in our 'fallen state', we may recognise that some humans require more protection because of their vulnerability rather than an imagined or romanticised innocence. It is because of our status as fallen creatures that we must take special care to protect the vulnerable in order to ensure that the strong do not rationalise their exploitation of the weak.

● ●

Susan and Thomas have a five-year-old daughter with a rare and life-threatening blood disorder. Her only hope for recovery is a blood or bone marrow transfusion, but no suitable donor can be found. One possibility would be to produce a second child who could provide suitable stem cells or bone marrow. This would entail using IVF and PGD in order to screen and select embryos that would be both free of the disorder and be compatible donors. Susan and Thomas want to have a second child, and wonder if they should pursue this option in order to 'save' their ill daughter as well. What advice would you offer Susan and Thomas? Why?

Postscript

THE PRIMARY PURPOSE of this book was to examine how theology might inform our deliberation on the morality of reproductive technology. Such theological themes as the vindicated order of creation, life as God's 'gift' and 'loan', our status as embodied creatures, and the natural and covenantal qualities of familial belonging were used in developing a framework of procreative stewardship. Within this framework a normative account of the parent–child relationship was sketched out in terms of certain vocations, virtues and practices that provide a familial setting of mutual and timely belonging. Various reproductive techniques were in turn assessed in respect to how they may either assist or impede prospective parents in preparing themselves to receive the gift of a child entrusted by God to their care.

A secondary purpose was to demonstrate an alternative mode of moral deliberation to that of procreative liberty. Thus developing a framework of procreative stewardship also served as an experiment to see how a moral assessment of reproductive technology might be shaped if attention were switched from the procedural issues of the rights and interests of autonomous persons to the biological, social and normative dimensions of familial bonds.

A systematic presentation of the book's theological and moral claims is beyond the scope of this limited exercise. Undertaking this more ambitious project would have resulted in a far different (as well as far larger) book, entailing a more extensive and detailed development of the principal theological themes and moral arguments. Such a book, however, would also fail to serve as an introductory text, suggesting ways in which theology might inform the reader's moral perception and assessment of reproductive technology. More modestly, my intention has been to indicate that alternative moral frameworks are available for shaping our perception and assessment of a growing capacity to control how life is passed on from one generation to the next. Thus this book was also written as an invitation to open and chart new avenues of further exploration.

These explorations are needed because of the extensive advances in reproductive technology, particularly in respect to quality control, now envisioned. Over the next few decades an unprecedented range of preventive and therapeutic treatments will be developed. One side effect of this progress, however, may be a diminished capacity to endure or tolerate suffering. As we come to believe that more and more diseases, disabilities and physical and behavioural limitations can be prevented, the category of 'unnecessary' suffering will enlarge. Why should someone endure physical pain or emotional distress if it is within our power to prevent the genetic factors contributing to the unwanted condition? Why keep company with the suffering if they serve to remind us of our failure to correct our biological deficiencies? In practical terms, children born with severe congenital defects may become increasingly stigmatised because their plight is preventable. In addition, their parents may be held accountable, if not morally or criminally culpable, for failing to prevent such unnecessary suffering.

This does not imply that suffering is inherently good. We should not allow people to suffer, or inflict suffering on others, to help build their character. Rather, there is a more tacit admission at stake that given the gift and grace of community, there are times when enduring suffering for our own or the sake of others is explicable. It is for the sake of these larger values and relationships that we may be called to suffer for or with others. Within this larger context the purpose of medicine is to help us live the type of lives we believe to be good, and right, and true. In pursuing such a life, suffering is not something we seek, but neither is it to be avoided at all cost. When medicine becomes fixated on avoiding suffering it not only corrupts itself as a healing art and moral community, but also has a corrupting influence on larger human relationships, such as the one between parent and child.

The obvious rejoinder to these fears is that future generations will live longer, healthier and more productive lives. What better gifts could be given to offspring? Yet will these qualities be conceived as gifts, or as the anticipated dividends of our reproductive investments? If it is the latter, then the cost will be to place a heavy burden on offspring, for they must simultaneously be an object of hope and the means of their parents' self-fulfilment. In fashioning children in an image and likeness of what their commissioners want them to become, they also personify the goal of what their progenitors are willing their future to be.

This goal, however, is a projection and magnification of ourselves, so it is through children that our dreams and aspirations are fulfilled. Our children are not so much like us, as artefacts created by and for us. This is one reason why Augustine argued against the notion that the birth of any child, save one, can ever be a proper object of hope. The future is not simply an extended and improved version of the present. We live instead in the hope of a destiny that awaits us. Children are properly regarded as gifts entrusted to the care of parents, for together they share the gift of a common destiny and grace rather than the task of constructing both.

Our growing capability to manipulate the human reproductive process and its outcomes may also reinforce a perception of both our individual lives and corporate life as projects to be undertaken instead of gifts to be safeguarded. 'Project' is an apt image for our age. We tend to believe that life is largely what we make of it. We create our lifestyles, we sculpt our bodies, and we make babies. We are contemplating the development of even more sophisticated reproductive technologies in a social context where children are becoming regarded as tools in fashioning our personal lives. If quality control techniques become widely deployed, it will be difficult to dismiss a prevalent notion of parental proprietorship over offspring.

If life is a gift, however, we cannot own children, because our lives are not our own. We are creatures who belong to God, and we belong with other creatures created in God's image and likeness. The metaphor of 'life as gift' should not be pressed too far, given its inherent limitations, but it does offer countervailing imagery to the equally distorting metaphor of 'life as project'.

If we perceive children as gifts entrusted to our care rather than outcomes of our reproductive projects, we confront a different set of concerns in developing and applying various reproductive technologies. If children are gifts, does this not imply a given and gratuitous structure to the parent–child relationship that is not subject to one's wilful manipulation? And if children are not properly a means of one's self-fulfilment, then does this not suggest an unconditional quality to the parent–child relationship that is not premised upon offspring possessing desirable traits?

My principal concern is that much of the moral inquiry accompanying the development of reproductive technology has fixated on questions of safety, efficacy and access. We may fail to take into account a matrix of subtle, though highly influential, cultural factors and expectations. For example, a widening range of quality-control techniques is being introduced at the very time when we are growing increasingly uncertain about what it means to be a parent or a child. This is witnessed by the awkward vocabulary we are concocting to describe our present circumstances. We now engage in 'parenting', suggesting that parents are adults who do something to children, rather than sharing a unique bond and unconditional relationship. With the technological advances we are now contemplating we will be able to do quite a lot to the bodies, minds and souls of children. As we exert greater qualitative control over the outcomes of our reproductive projects, will we come to see offspring simply as young people 'childing' in response to their 'parenting'? This is a not a fanciful or alarmist spectre. We already casually talk about investing in our children's future by obtaining the best education, activities and gadgets money can buy. Why not add a genetic endowment to the list?

It needs to be emphasised that the issue at stake is not reproductive technology per se. Individually many current applications, as well as new technologies envisioned, promote more effective and humane medical treatments. It is the cumulative effect of these developments, however, that should give us some pause. As each new technology is placed in forming a larger pattern, the moral landscape is also altered. As new technological advances are introduced, our perceptions and expectations regarding longevity, health, autonomy, familial relationships, community and the ordering of larger human associations will change accordingly. Although a more expansive use of reproductive technology may not result in either our best dreams or worst nightmares, we should at least acknowledge that they will transform the course of our moral deliberation on what constitutes a good life and how it should be pursued.

This is why our further steps towards controlling human reproduction should also be accompanied by fresh theological explorations, prompting a fundamental moral debate. We need to be aware of the beliefs and hopes that are driving our reproductive projects, and to assess their veracity and efficacy accordingly. Moreover, this public debate needs to be initiated in a manner ensuring that the subsequent reshaping of the moral landscape is prompted more by deliberate conviction than by the sheer force of technological capability and efficiency. In short, it is one thing to ponder the prospect of reproductive technology as an instrument enabling our procreative stewardship, and quite another to see it as a tool for constructing and mastering our fate.

Notes

Introduction
1. 'New families for old?' in Carole Ulanowsky (ed.), *The Family in the Age of Biotechnology* (Aldershot: Avebury, 1995), p.28.
2. See 1 Corinthians 13:9–12.

Chapter 1: **Reproductive Options**
1. Psalm 139.13–14 (NRSV).
2. For further descriptions and statistical summaries of assisted techniques used in the UK and US, consult the Human Fertilisation and Embryology Authority (*www.hfea.gov.uk*), the American Society for Reproductive Medicine (*www.asrm.org*), and the Centers for Disease Control and Prevention, section on Reproductive Health Information Sources (*www.cdc.gov/nccdphp/drh*).
3. See, e.g., Deuteronomy 25:5–6.
4. An amniocentesis is usually performed between the fifteenth and sixteenth week of pregnancy.
5. CVS is usually performed between the ninth and eleventh weeks of pregnancy.
6. Michael Burgess, 'The medicalization of dying', *The Journal of Medicine and Philosophy* 18 (June 1993), 270–1.
7. See, for example, Anne Borrowdale, *Reconstructing Family Values* (London: SPCK, 1994), and Christine E. Gudorf, *Body, Sex, and Pleasure: Reconstructing Christian sexual ethics* (Cleveland, Ohio: Pilgrim Press, 1994).
8. Marilyn Strathern, *Reproducing the Future: Essays on anthropology, kinship and the new reproductive technologies* (Manchester: Manchester University Press, 1992), p. 30.
9. See Barbara Katz Rothman, *The Tentative Pregnancy: Amniocentesis and the sexual politics of motherhood* (London: Pandora, 1994); see also Elizabeth Kristol, 'Picture perfect: the politics of prenatal testing', *First Things*, 32 (April 1993), 17–24.
10. See John Robertson *Children of Choice: Freedom and the new reproductive technologies* (Princeton, New Jersey: Princeton University Press, 1994).
11. Ibid., p. 22.
12. Ibid., p. 24.
13. Ibid., p. 35.
14. Ibid., p. 100.
15. It is difficult to discern how this intermediate position treats embryos with any greater respect than that afforded to human tissue. See Gilbert Meilaender, *Bioethics: A primer for Christians* (Grand Rapids, Michigan: Eerdmans, 1996), pp. 109–13.
16. Robertson, *Children of Choice*, pp. 119–45.
17. Ibid., p. 126.

18. Ibid., p. 131.
19. Ibid., p. 172.
20. Ibid., p. 167.
21. Ibid., p. 145.
22. Robert Song, *Christianity and Liberal Society* (Oxford: Clarendon Press, 1997), p. 9. See also pp. 9–48.
23. H. Tristram Engelhardt, *The Foundations of Bioethics* (New York and Oxford: Oxford University Press, 1996).
24. See ibid., pp. 3–4.
25. See ibid., pp. 74–8.
26. Ibid., p. 120 (emphasis added).
27. Ibid., p. 139.
28. See ibid., pp. 149–51.
29. Ibid., p. 149.

Chapter 2: **Theological Themes**
1. See Karl Barth, *Church Dogmatics* III/4 (Edinburgh: T. & T. Clark, 1961), pp. 327–8.
2. See Genesis 2:7.
3. See Barth, *Church Dogmatics* III/4, pp. 329–32.
4. See Genesis 1:24–8.
5. See Oliver O'Donovan, *Resurrection and Moral Order* (Leicester: Inter-Varsity Press, 1986), pp. 31–52.
6. See ibid., pp. 13–15.
7. Ibid., p. 122.
8. Paul Ramsey, *One Flesh: A Christian view of sex within, outside and before marriage* (Bramcote: Grove Books, 1975), p. 4.
9. See *City of God* XXII.
10. See Genesis 1:31.
11. See Romans 8:18–25.
12. See Barth, *Church Dogmatics* III/4, pp. 116–17; cf. Emil Brunner, *The Divine Imperative* (London: Lutterworth Press, 1937), pp. 347–9.
13. See Rodney Clapp, *Families at the Crossroads: Beyond traditional and modern options* (Leicester: Inter-Varsity Press, 1993), pp. 125–8.
14. See *One Flesh*, pp. 4–14.
15. Paul Ramsey, *Fabricated Man: The ethics of genetic control* (New Haven, Connecticut and London: Yale University Press, 1970), pp. 38–9 (emphasis original).
16. Ramsey, *One Flesh*, p. 13.
17. See Stanley Hauerwas, *Suffering Presence: Theological reflections on medicine, the mentally handicapped, and the church* (Notre Dame, Indiana: University of Notre Dame Press, 1986), pp. 148–52, and *A Community of Character: Toward a constructive Christian ethic* (Notre Dame, Indiana and London: University of Notre Dame Press, 1981), pp. 168–74.
18. See Robertson, *Children of Choice*, pp. 119–45.
19. Gilbert C. Meilaender, *Body, Soul, and Bioethics* (Notre Dame, Indiana and London: University of Notre Dame Press, 1995), p. 88.
20. See Oliver O'Donovan, *Begotten or Made?* (Oxford: Clarendon Press, 1984), pp. 1–13.
21. Ramsey, *Fabricated Man*, p. 34.

Chapter 3: **Childlessness and Parenthood**

1. See John Rogerson, 'The family and structures of grace in the Old Testament' in Stephen C. Barton (ed.), *The Family in Theological Perspective* (Edinburgh: T. & T. Clark, 1996), pp. 43–64; and Stephen C. Barton, 'The relativisation of family ties in the Jewish and Graeco-Roman traditions' in Halvor Moxnes (ed.), *Constructing Early Christian Families: Family as social reality and metaphor* (London and New York: Routledge, 1997), pp. 81–100.
2. Santiago Guijarro, 'The family in first-century Galilee' in Moxnes (ed.), *Constructing Early Christian Families*, p. 43.
3. See ibid., pp. 48–9.
4. See ibid., pp. 57–61; see also Beryl Rawson, 'The Roman family' in Beryl Rawson (ed.), *The Family in Ancient Rome: New perspectives* (London: Routledge, 1992), pp. 8–15.
5. John Barclay, 'The family as the bearer of religion in Judaism and early Christianity' in Moxnes (ed.), *Constructing Early Christian Families*, p. 69.
6. See Rawson, 'The Roman family' in Rawson (ed.), *The Family in Ancient Rome*, pp. 15–31.
7. Peter Brown, *The Body and Society: Men, women, and sexual renunciation in early Christianity* (New York: Columbia University Press, 1988), p. 6.
8. See Matthew 19:3–12 and Mark 10:2–12.
9. See Matthew 19:13–15, Mark 10:13–16 and Luke 18:16–18.
10. See Barclay, 'The family as the bearer of religion in Judaism and Early Christianity' in Moxnes (ed.), *Constructing Early Christian Families*, pp. 72–7.
11. Ibid., p. 73.
12. Ibid., p. 74.
13. See 1 Corinthians 7.
14. See Stephen Barton, 'Paul's sense of place: an anthropological approach to community formation in Corinth', *New Testament Studies* 32 (1986), 225–46.
15. Don S. Browning et al., *From Culture Wars to Common Ground: Religion and the American family debate* (Louisville, Kentucky: Westminster John Knox Press, 1997), p. 136.
16. See Colossians 3:18—4:1; Ephesians 5:22—6:9; 1 Peter 2:18—3:7; 1 Timothy 2:8–15; 6:1–2; and Titus 2:1–10.
17. James Dunn, 'The household rules in the New Testament' in Barton (ed.), *The Family in Theological Perspective*, p. 48.
18. Carol Harrison, 'The silent majority: the family in patristic thought' in Barton (ed.), *The Family in Theological Perspective*, p. 87.
19. *Miscellanies* III/46.
20. See *Concerning Virgins* I/64.
21. See *On Virginity* III.
22. See ibid. XIII.
23. See *On Exhortation to Chastity* XII.
24. See *On Marriage and Concupiscence* I/8.
25. See Paul Ramsey, 'Human sexuality in the history of redemption', *The Journal of Religious Ethics* 16:1 (Spring 1988), 66.
26. See Augustine, *Of Holy Virginity* XVIII.
27. See Thomas Aquinas, *Summa Theologiae* (Supplement) XLI.
28. See *The Judgment of Martin Luther on Monastic Vows* in James Atkinson (ed.), *Luther's Works* Vol. 44 (Philadelphia, Pennsylvania: Fortress Press, 1966), pp. 245–400.
29. See Martin Luther, *The Estate of Marriage* in Walter I. Brandt (ed.), *Luther's Works* Vol. 45 (Philadelphia: Muhlenberg Press, 1962), pp. 17ff.

30. See Richard Baxter, *A Christian Directory, Part II: Christian economics (or family duties)* Vol. 4 of the *Practical Works* (London: James Duncan, 1830).
31. F. D. Maurice, *Social Morality: Twenty-one lectures delivered in the University of Cambridge* (London and Cambridge: Macmillan & Co., 1869).
32. See Horace Bushnell, *Christian Nurture* (New Haven, Connecticut: Yale University Press, 1947).
33. See Gilbert C. Meilaender, *Bioethics: A Primer for Christians* (Grands Rapids, Michigan: Eerdmans, 1996), pp. 13–15.
34. See *Donum Vitae* II.
35. See Germain Grisez, *The Way of the Lord Jesus* II (Quincy, Illinois: Franciscan Press, 1993), pp. 569–74.
36. See ibid., p. 689.
37. See Lisa Sowle Cahill, *Sex, Gender, and Christian Ethics* (Cambridge: Cambridge University Press, 1996), pp. 217–54.
38. See Christine E. Gudorf, *Body, Sex, and Pleasure: Reconstructing Christian sexual ethics* (Cleveland, Ohio: Pilgrim Press, 1994), pp. 29–50.
39. See D. Gareth Jones, *Manufacturing Humans: The challenge of the new reproductive technologies* (Leicester: Inter-Varsity Press, 1987), pp. 240–69; James Gustafson, *Ethics from a Theocentric Perspective* I (Chicago and London: University of Chicago Press, 1981), pp. 281–93, and 'A Protestant ethical approach' in S. E. Lammers and A. Verhey (eds), *On Moral Medicine: Theological perspectives in medical ethics* (Grand Rapids, Michigan and Cambridge: Eerdmans, 1998), pp. 403–12; Anthony Dyson, *The Ethics of IVF* (London and New York: Mowbray, 1995), pp. 108–20.
40. See Ted Peters, *For the Love of Children: Genetic technology and the future of the family* (Louisville, Kentucky: Westminster John Knox Press, 1996), pp. 40–84.
41. Grisez, *The Way of the Lord Jesus* II, p. 690.
42. Ibid.
43. See *Sex, Gender, and Christian Ethics*, pp. 246–9.
44. Ibid., p. 247.
45. Ibid.
46. Ibid.
47. Ibid., p. 249.
48. Peters, *For the Love of Children*, p. 32.
49. Ibid., p. 12.
50. Oliver O'Donovan, *Begotten or Made?* (Oxford: Clarendon Press, 1984), p. 35.
51. Ibid., p. 37.
52. Ibid.
53. See John A. Robertson, *Children of Choice: Freedom and the new reproductive technologies* (Princeton, New Jersey: Princeton University Press, 1994), pp. 142–4.
54. See Grisez, *The Way of the Lord Jesus* II, p. 569.
55. Meilaender, *Bioethics*, p. 24.
56. Ibid., p. 25.

Chapter 4: **Preventing and Assisting Reproduction**

1. Gilbert C. Meilaender, *Body, Soul, and Bioethics* (Notre Dame, Indiana and London: University of Notre Dame Press, 1995), p. 84 (emphasis added).
2. *Humanae Vitae* V/3.
3. Ibid. V/1.
4. Ibid. V/9.
5. See ibid. V/14.

6. See Charles Curran, 'Natural law and contemporary moral theology' in Charles Curran (ed.), *Contraception: Authority and dissent* (London: Burns & Oates, 1969).

7. See Karl Rahner, 'On the Encyclical "Humanae Vitae"' in *Theological Investigations* XI (London: Darton, Longman & Todd, 1974).

8. See Bernard Haering, 'The inseparability of the unitive-procreative functions of the marital act' in Curran (ed.), *Contraception: Authority and dissent*.

9. See Bernard Haering, 'The Encyclical crisis' in Daniel Callahan (ed.), *The Catholic Case for Contraception* (London: Arlington Books, 1969).

10. See Richard McCormick, *How Brave a New World? Dilemmas in bioethics* (London: SCM Press, 1981), pp. 221–4, and *Health and Medicine in the Catholic Tradition: Tradition in transition* (New York: Crossroad, 1984), pp. 92–9.

11. See Sidney Callahan, 'Procreation and control' in Callahan (ed.), *The Catholic Case for Contraception*.

12. See Janet E. Smith, *Humanae Vitae: A generation later* (Washington DC: Catholic University of America Press, 1991), pp. 85–6.

13. See ibid., 118–28.

14. See Germain Grisez, *The Way of the Lord Jesus* II (Quincy, Illinois: Franciscan Press, 1993), pp. 507–12.

15. *Donum Vitae*, Foreword.

16. Ibid., Introduction/2.

17. Ibid., Introduction/4.

18. See Grisez, *The Way of the Lord Jesus* II, pp. 267–8, 684.

19. See Stanley Hauerwas, *Suffering Presence: Theological reflections on medicine, the mentally handicapped, and the church* (Notre Dame Indiana: University of Notre Dame Press, 1986), pp. 144–52.

20. See Oliver O'Donovan, *Begotten or Made?* (Oxford: Clarendon Press, 1984), pp. 31–66.

21. See Thomas Shannon and Lisa Sowle Cahill, *Religion and Artificial Reproduction: An inquiry into the Vatican 'Instruction on Respect for Human Life in its Origin and on the Dignity of Human Reproduction'* (New York: Crossroad, 1988), pp. 103–32.

22. See Paul Ramsey *Fabricated Man: The ethics of genetic control* (New Haven, Connecticut and London: Yale University Press, 1970). pp. 112, 138; and 'Shall we reproduce? I: The medical ethics of *in vitro* fertilization', *Journal of the American Medical Association* 220 (1972), 1346–50.

23. See McCormick, *How Brave a New World?*, pp. 321–33.

24. See Karl Rahmer 'The problem of genetic manipulation' in *Theological Investigations* IX (London: Darton, Longman & Todd, 1972), pp. 243–51.

25. See Sidney Callahan, 'Lovemaking and babymaking: ethics and the new reproductive technology', *Commonweal* (24 April 1987), 233–9.

26. See Charles Curran, 'Theology and genetics: a multi-faceted dialogue', *Journal of Ecumenical Studies* 7 (1970), 61–89.

27. See James Gustafson, 'Basic ethical issues in the biomedical fields', *Soundings* 53 (1970), 151–80.

28. See D. Gareth Jones, *Manufacturing Humans: The challenge of the new reproductive technologies* (Leicester: Inter-Varsity Press, 1987), pp. 240–64.

29. See Ted Peters, *For the Love of Children: Genetic technology and the future of the family* (Louisville, Kentucky: Westminster John Knox Press, 1996), pp. 40–84.

30. George Grant, *English-Speaking Justice* (Notre Dame, Indiana: University of Notre Dame Press, 1985), p. 82.

31. See George Grant, *Technology and Justice* (Notre Dame, Indiana: University of Notre Dame Press, 1986), p. 12.
32. Ibid., p. 19; see also pp. 19–28.
33. Ibid., p. 32.
34. Ibid.
35. Ibid.
36. See John A. Robertson, *Children of Choice: Freedom and the new reproductive technologies* (Princeton, New Jersey: Princeton University Press, 1994), pp. 234–5.
37. Meilaender, *Body, Soul, and Bioethics*, p. 87.

Chapter 5: **Quality Control and Experimentation**

1. See HFEA, *Consultation Document on Preimplantation Genetic Diagnosis*, Annex C, 3.2.1–3.3.1.
2. See ibid., Annex C, 3.3.3.
3. See ibid., Section A, 3–6.
4. See ibid., Section A, 1.
5. See ibid., Section B, 14–19.
6. See ibid., Section B, 20–35.
7. See ibid., Section C, 36–8.
8. See ibid., Section C, 39–47.
9. See HFEA Code of Practice (fourth edition, July 1998), Chapter 10.
10. See John A. Robertson, *Children of Choice: Freedom and the new reproductive technologies* (Princeton, New Jersey: Princeton University Press, 1994), pp. 170–1.
11. See *Donum Vitae* I/2, and Germain Grisez, *The Way of the Lord Jesus* II (Quincy, Illinois: Franciscan Press, 1993), pp. 489–98, 504.
12. See Paul Ramsey, *Fabricated Man: The ethics of genetic control* (New Haven, Connecticut and London: Yale University Press, 1970), pp. 130–38.
13. See D. Gareth Jones, *Manufacturing Humans: The challenge of the new reproductive technologies* (Leicester: Inter-Varsity Press, 1987), pp. 125–67.
14. See James Gustafson, *Ethics from a Theocentric Perspective* I (Chicago and London: University of Chicago Press, 1981), pp. 281–93, and 'A Protestant ethical approach' in S. E. Lammers and A. Verhey (eds), *On Moral Medicine: Theological perspectives on medical ethics* (Grand Rapids, Michigan and Cambridge: Eerdmans, 1998), pp. 600–11.
15. See Joseph Fletcher, *The Ethics of Genetic Control* (Garden City, New York: Anchor Books, 1974), pp. 147–87, and 'Four indicators of humanhood – the enquiry matters', *Hastings Center Report* 4 (December 1975), 4–7.
16. See Stanley Hauerwas, *Suffering Presence: Theological reflections on medicine, the mentally handicapped, and the church* (Notre Dame, Indiana: University of Notre Dame Press, 1986), pp. 63–83; see also *Naming the Silences: God, medicine, and the problem of suffering* (Grand Rapids, Michigan: Eerdmans, 1990), pp. 1–38.
17. See Hauerwas, *Suffering Presence*, pp. 39–62.
18. See Ronald Cole-Turner and Brent Waters, *Pastoral Genetics: Theology and care at the beginning of life* (Cleveland, Ohio: Pilgrim Press, 1996), pp. 57–65.
19. See Ronald Cole-Turner, 'Do means matter?' and Eric Juengst, 'What does enhancement mean?' in Erik Parens (ed.), *Enhancing Human Traits: Ethical and social implications* (Washington DC: Georgetown University Press, 1998).
20. For discussions concerning what these circumstances encompass, see Oliver O'Donovan, *The Christian and the Unborn Child* (Bramcote: Grove Books,

1973), pp. 17–21, and Gilbert Meilaender, *Bioethics: A primer for Christians* (Grand Rapids, Michigan: Eerdmans, 1996), pp. 26–38.

21. See Oliver O'Donovan, 'Again: who is a person?' in J. H. Channer (ed.), *Abortion and the Sanctity of Human Life* (Exeter: Paternoster Press, 1985), p. 129 (emphasis original).

Glossary

Amniocentesis: A technique examining fetal cells from the amniotic fluid surrounding a fetus. The cells are tested for genetic or chromosomal abnormalities.

Assisted Reproductive Technologies (ART): A shorthand reference to techniques assisting the fertilisation of an oocyte or egg either within or outside a woman's body.

Chorionic Villus Sampling (CVS): A technique for removing a small sample of placental tissue that is tested for genetic abnormalities.

Cloning: Techniques (nuclear transfer or embryo splitting) creating genetically identical individuals.

Collaborative Reproduction: Techniques requiring donated gametes and/or surrogacy. Some collaborative arrangements may include gamete donors or surrogates providing parental care following birth.

Embryo: A fertilised egg up to the eighth week of development.

Fetus: An embryo after the eighth week of development.

Gamete: Female egg or male sperm.

Gamete Intrafallopian Transfer (GIFT): A technique in which eggs are mixed with sperm and then placed in a woman's fallopian tube so that fertilisation may occur within a woman's body.

Human Fertilisation and Embryology Authority (HFEA): Regulatory agency in the United Kingdom overseeing the use of reproductive technologies, and experimentation involving embryos.

Human Genome Project (HGP): International research project to map and sequence the human genetic code.

In Vitro Fertilisation (IVF): A technique for fertilising eggs outside a woman's body.

Laparoscopy: A surgical procedure for examining the pelvic cavity. An incision is made below the navel, and a small optical instrument is inserted.

Preimplantation Genetic Diagnosis (PGD): Genetically testing an embryo prior to implantation in a woman's uterus.

Prenatal Diagnosis (PND): The screening or testing of embryos or fetuses for chromosomal or genetic abnormalities.

Quality Control: A shorthand phrase referring to techniques designed to prevent the birth of a severely ill or disabled child. These techniques may also be used to prevent the birth of children with undesirable characteristics, or to select in favour of desirable characteristics.

Surrogacy: A woman providing gestation, usually for a couple in which the woman is unable to conceive or maintain a pregnancy. The surrogate may be genetically related to the child she carries if artificial insemination is used, or genetically unrelated if ZIFT is used.

Zygote Intrafallopian Transfer (ZIFT): A zygote or fertilised egg is placed in a woman's fallopian tube.

Select Annotated Bibliography

Brown, Peter. *The Body and Society: Men, women, and sexual renunciation in early Christianity*. New York: Columbia University Press, 1988. A comprehensive overview of early Christian attitudes on singleness, marriage and family.

Callahan, Daniel (ed.). *The Catholic Case for Contraception*. London: Arlington Books, 1969. An anthology of Catholic authors arguing in favour of contraception.

Cahill, Lisa Sowle. *Sex, Gender, and Christian Ethics*. Cambridge: Cambridge University Press, 1996. Written from both a Catholic and feminist perspective, this book argues that sex, commitment and parenthood are essential elements in forging crucial human relationships.

Chadwick, Ruth F. (ed.). *Ethics, Reproduction and Genetic Control* (revised edn). London and New York: Routledge, 1992. A collection of articles that introduce and discuss a wide range of topics and issues.

Cole-Turner, Ronald, and Waters, Brent. *Pastoral Genetics: Theology and care at the beginning of life*. Cleveland, Ohio: Pilgrim Press, 1996. Examines a wide variety of quality-control issues from a pastoral perspective.

Gudorf, Christine E. *Body, Sex, and Pleasure: Reconstructing Christian sexual ethics*. Cleveland, Ohio: Pilgrim Press, 1994. A feminist critique of traditional Christian views on sex, procreation, marriage and family.

Harris, John. *Clones, Genes, and Immortality: Ethics and the genetic revolution*. Oxford and New York: Oxford University Press, 1998. A philosophical argument opposing restrictions upon assisted reproductive technologies or quality control techniques.

Hauerwas, Stanley. *Suffering Presence: Theological reflections on medicine, the mentally handicapped, and the church*. Notre Dame, Indiana: University of Notre Dame Press, 1986. A theological analysis of prevalent attitudes on medicine, illness and suffering.

Lammers, Stephen E., and Verhey, Allen (eds). *On Moral Medicine: Theological perspectives in medical ethics* (second edn). Grand Rapids, Michigan, and Cambridge: Eerdmans, 1998. A comprehensive anthology of both critical and constructive articles on contemporary medicine. The sections focusing on various aspects of procreation and human agency provide an especially helpful introduction.

Meilaender, Gilbert C. *Body, Soul, and Bioethics*. Notre Dame, Indiana, and London: University of Notre Dame Press, 1995. A theological reflection on how reproductive technology is exerting a fragmenting influence on how procreation and parenthood are coming to be perceived. Includes an extended critique of Robertson's 'procreative liberty'.

O'Donovan, Oliver. *Begotten or Made?* Oxford: Clarendon Press, 1984. A theological argument against reproductive technology on the basis that it disrupts a relationship of fundamental equality between parents and offspring, thereby transforming children into artefacts.

O'Donovan, Oliver. *Resurrection and Moral Order: An outline for evangelical ethics*.

Leicester: Inter-Varsity Press, 1986. Provides many of the foundational arguments underlying the account of procreative stewardship presented in this book.

Peters, Ted. *For the Love of Children: Genetic technology and the future of the family.* Louisville, Kentucky: Westminster John Knox Press, 1996. Argues that various reproductive technologies are permissible so long as they enable parents to express a fundamental and overriding love for children.

Ramsey, Paul. *Fabricated Man: The ethics of genetic control.* New Haven, Connecticut and London: Yale University Press, 1970. An early assessment of the ethics of reproductive technology, especially in regard to quality-control issues.

Ramsey, Paul. *One Flesh: A Christian view of sex within, outside and before marriage.* Bramcote: Grove Books, 1975. Argues on behalf of a normative structure ordering the relationship among marriage, procreation and parenthood.

Robertson, John A. *Children of Choice: Freedom and the new reproductive technologies.* Princeton, New Jersey: Princeton University Press, 1994. A philosophical presentation of the basic principles underlying procreative liberty or reproductive freedom.

Index